Guilty
Prayers

Guilty Prayers

Do you have issues with anger, bitterness, guilt, or depression?

Read the individual stories about people who let these emotions get out of control. Learn what they did to resolve the devastating outcomes from emotions gone wild.

JANET LYNAS, PHD, NHD

For information about this title or to order other books and/or electronic media,
contact the publisher:

Mind-Body Connection Hypnosis
jlhypnosisthreapy@gmail.com

ISBNs
Print: 978-0-578-49610-8
eBook: 978-0-578-49885-0

Printed in the United States of America

Cover and Interior design: 1106 Design

To my mentor and friend, Starr

*This book is completed because of your faith in me.
Every time I sit down to write I hear, "More adjectives!
More sparkles!" These words echo in my sleep as well.*

*You have pushed me to reach new heights both in my
writing and in my personal life. You have pushed me to the
point of frustration at times, which is what I needed.*

*My deepest gratitude,
Janet*

Contents

Introduction

Guilty Prayers was penned (literally penned) over thirty years ago. It started out as an article for publication with a Christian magazine. But as life often does, it threw me a curve. The story was packed away for a move as I transitioned from one community to another. Three moves and thirty-two years later, it was found in the bottom of a file cabinet drawer.

Each chapter is based on a true story with the people who were involved telling their own story and the struggles they had in dealing with their emotions. I have taken their stories and expanded each one to address what happens if we do not face the challenges that come our way as we journey through life.

As I have matured, so has Guilty Prayers. You will find a common theme throughout this book. The first lesson is to pay attention to what you are thinking. We are what we think and we manifest into our lives what we think. If you think, "I am poor," then so you shall be.

The second lesson you will find in this book is to know yourself. Until you know who you truly are, you will not be able to have a meaningful and deep relationship with your Creator or with anyone else. It is scary to take a look at the dark shadow side of our emotions. It is deep within these shadows that we do not want to look because we do not want to admit that we have this dark side. This shadow side of ourselves makes us tremble in fear, because we do not want to admit to ourselves that we could possibly have such dark thoughts and tendencies.

Guilty Prayers, we all pray them. How do we work through life's crises? What happens if we do not? Guilty Prayers takes a look at guilt, bitterness, fear, emotional pain, self-blame, depression, lost love, forgiveness, prayers, getting to know God, and judging. All of these emotions are detrimental to us mentally, physically, emotionally, and spiritually if not acknowledged and dealt with.

It is by no chance or oversight that Guilty Prayers has thirteen chapters. The number thirteen in Angle numbers represents a message from your angels that some upheavals may take place in your life. This is just what happened to me.

In June of 2012, I was diagnosed with melanoma, I went through a divorce, sold my house that I had lived in for eighteen years, bought a new house in my hometown, and moved back to my childhood community to be close to family again. It was time to go home.

August 4, 2017, I was run over by a semitruck. My car was totaled and I received a concussion causing a headache that has been with me every day since the accident, which at this time has been over a year. I was not able to return to my nursing career because of the headache and occasional brain fog. I lost a vital part of who I am that day. Nursing was not a job or career for me, but a passion and my mission in serving people.

Angel number thirteen also means that the upheaval can be a blessing in disguise. That is certainly true in my case. Spirit has been nudging me all these years to write articles and books that will help people and bless their lives. In past years, I have been published in magazines and papers, however, it was only occasionally that I wrote. This is not what Creator God wanted from me.

Angel number thirteen is also a message that my angels and ascended masters are guiding me and helping me along my life's journey. I know this to be true for me. The semitruck running over my car was not caused by my slow movement to transition into the life that my God had been asking me to do for years. But, the situation was used to help me learn that all my needs would be met, even when I was unsure where the money was coming from to pay my bills. My needs have always been met by my angels and Creator. I am now living my Divine purpose and helping people in a different way. I am following my Divine path. I learned how to step out on faith and truly trust God to show me that I AM always cared for and Loved.

When I was a little girl, my mother told me I used to say, "Come on, Jesus, let's go play." That is just what I am doing now. Jesus and I are having a great time playing.

It is my sincerest and deepest prayer that you will find Guilty Prayers a blessing for your life.

So it is said, and so it is done. Blessings to you.

1

Guilty Prayers

BY

JANET LYNAS

"God, why won't she die? I can't take this anymore! Don't you care whether or not she hurts? Can't you hear her screaming out in pain? God, if you are not going to heal her, then let her die. Or, do you like seeing her suffer like this?"

Guilty Prayers, we all pray them. What causes the conflict in our prayer life? Do we become a sinner when we utter prayers of strife?

We come to a crossroads and wonder how should we pray? A wife, husband, child, or someone we hold dear becomes terminally ill, or fate deals a cruel blow and someone is hurt beyond human repair. Our hearts are torn in crushing, anguished pain and we do not know how to pray. Do we pray that they will be spared from this horrible suffering? Do we pray for prolonged life? What are we supposed to pray and how do we pray?

We do not want to see our loved one in this agonizing pain. Suffering is an ugly sight, the pain is gut-wrenching and unbearable to watch. We do not know how to deal with life's harsh realities. It is hard to accept the fact that life is fragile and easily broken. We feel uncomfortable praying for this person's needs because we really do not know what their needs are. If we should pray, why? If we pray for the suffering to stop, we feel like we are wishing our loved one dead. We want the suffering to stop, but we are afraid to pray, we become paralyzed with fear, uncertain of the fear within our own weaknesses. We cry out to God Almighty with hearts broken in agony begging Him to put a stop to this vicious attack on our loved one. Our tears flowing freely, as we cry out in sorrowful pain from our broken heart pleading for an intervention.

Life is precious. We want to extend life into old age. We can't let our loved one die, especially if the years have been few. Life has to be supported until a healing from God or man can take place. Life supports are hooked up and then, when the time comes, panic and terror rushes in when it is time to remove the tubes, fluids, and machines. Life has drained from the body, yet machines pump air into the lungs and fluids into the veins.

Worry creeps in once the machines are turned off, was that the right thing to do? The stillness in the room once the machines are turned off is more than we can endure; worry gives way to uncontrollable panic. The silence in the room, it is too much to bear; horror sets in and we suddenly find that we want the machines turned back on, but it is too late. Should we have left the machines running a little longer? Did we kill our loved one? Did we betray the trust they had in us? And, was their love that they had in us sold out? Reasoning powers have long deserted us. We can no longer understand that the broken body was beyond repair.

If the loss is a child, we not only mourn the child's death, but we mourn what their life might have been. We grieve who they may have become. We miss seeing our baby grow into adulthood, experiencing our child's marriage. And then seeing them become parents and having children of their own. We miss out on being grandparents to our baby's little ones. We dwell on what might have been. We promised our child that we would protect them no matter what might come their way when they were born. But, we failed to protect our child. We failed our little one. We failed as a parent. How could we have let our child die? We can't accept that, at times, circumstances may be beyond our control.

With the loss of a spouse, we find that our lifestyle has suddenly changed; children to rear alone and no one to give us support with the parenting responsibilities. There is little time to meet personal needs now that we have been thrown into a new way of living, a lifestyle of being a single parent. It is not an easy lifestyle. There are many lonely moments. There are challenges in dealing with stubborn children. You find that you are always wondering if you are making the right decisions as you are parenting your children. At times, you may feel like you are drowning in the responsibilities that come with being a single parent. You find that you are always second-guessing yourself. It is exhausting!

Steven found himself struggling with guilty prayers. "Patricia had complained after the birth of our second child that it felt like something was left inside of her," began Steven with a heaviness in his voice as he recalled the events.

After a few weeks of growing discomfort and pain Patricia sought medical help. She was given a proctoscopic examination and an antibiotic for an infection.

"About two months later she developed extremely severe stomach pains. Early one morning Patricia woke up screaming in excruciating pain. She was having stabbing pains in her stomach again that caused her to double over in tortured agony. This time she went to a different doctor," Steven continued. "The pain became so severe during the day that the doctor admitted her to the hospital. Tests were scheduled right away."

The test revealed gallstones and a blockage in her colon. Surgery was scheduled for the following week. Little did Patricia and Steven realize how serious her illness really was. They had no idea of the challenges that lay ahead of them. Least of all, they had no idea that time was limited and how quickly it would slip away.

"When the surgeon came out and said, 'I'm sorry, your wife has colon cancer. It's in the advanced stages.' I was stunned," Steven said, speaking slowly. "I walked in a dazed stupor for about two hours before I could call family members. I have no idea where I walked or what I was doing. Time stood still and faded into the background as I tried to comprehend what the doctor had just told me. She was only in her early thirties, how could she have advanced cancer? How can you comprehend that your wife is dying?"

Even though doctors gave Patricia and Steven no hope, a frantic search was started to find a cure for Patricia. Thousands of dollars were spent going from one doctor to another seeking a cure. Steven finally had to face facts, there was nothing he or the doctors could do.

"We tried health foods, radiation, chiropractors. We even went to Mexico," Steven recalled. "One doctor told us 'I don't know why you came to me. There's nothing I can do.' I was livid with his bluntness. His lack of compassion devastated Patricia."

Patricia's frantic search continued as she went from one religious denomination to another. Even though her condition worsened and she had to have gallbladder surgery just three months after the colon surgery, Patricia was convinced by faith healers that her faith had healed her. She was convinced that her cancer was gone.

We tend to overlook the impossibilities of God. He can't do anything that is bad or sinful. God's power is unlimited except by His own moral nature and by certain self-imposed limitations He has built into His world. The laws of restriction that Creator God adheres to will not allow Him to violate His own rules. We do not know all these laws; we are still discovering them. However, we do know these laws come out of the character of God the Creator and they express His inner stability.

I AM THAT I AM will not violate human freedom. He created us with the freedom to make choices. It is evident that His usual way of healing is to use the best of human knowledge and medical skills. He gave the command for man to have dominion over the earth and subdue it. Our Universal Life Force seems to wait for us to do just that and bring healing through a natural means. The exception is supernatural ways. The trouble is, when we try to make the exception the rule.

Eighteen months after the first surgery, Steven found himself spending more and more time at the hospital. Still, Patricia was convinced she was healed. She wrote to the *The 700 Club*, a Christian television show, to proclaim a healing from God. It was irrational for her to think that she was healed when follow-up tests showed that the cancer had spread throughout her body, but Patricia continued to proclaim that she was cancer free. She was frantically grasping at straws for a cure. She had no lifeline to hold on to, but still she was grasping for any thread of hope she could find. Patricia's fear had overtaken rational thinking. Her fear was out of control.

"I remember thinking, Lord God, why doesn't she just die? When will the screams from pain stop? She's a living corpse. I can't stand listening to the screaming anymore."

Then, when Patricia did die, Steven wondered if his prayers had killed her. Did he do all he could to save her? Logic had escaped him just as it had escaped Patricia.

"I could only wonder about 'What ifs. What if I had taken her to another doctor? What if we had tried another procedure? What if. . . ," Steven remembers.

Steven felt guilty at times and blamed himself for Patricia's death. He did not know newly widowed people frequently believe that they were not able to do enough to help their spouse during a prolonged illness or at the time of their death.

Steven's guilt deepened as he began to think his prayers had killed Patricia. His health began to suffer and to deteriorate from the guilt he carried within.

"Slowly, I became aware that I was wishing Patricia dead not only to relieve her pain, but also for my own convenience and release from stress," Steven said, hanging his head in shame.

The stress of Patricia's illness and death on Steven had aged him beyond his years, making him look old and weathered. The weight of the stress had taken a toll on Steven causing him to bend from the heaviness placed on his shoulders.

Every marital relationship has pain and disappointment. Most marriages have areas of unrest and anger. Steven and Patricia had had their problems during their marriage. Patricia had felt that Steven should spend every free moment with her; she became upset when he was doing maintenance on his truck. They argued about how time should be managed, about how money should be spent, and in the end about the faith healers telling her she was cured, that her cancer was gone.

It is normal for people to think at times, "If it were not for you I would be happy, adjusted, out-of-debt . . ." If there are harsh words or a disagreement prior to the death, the surviving spouse is often guilt-ridden because of an inability to undo the lingering bad feelings.

"I began to dwell on every single disagreement we had ever had," Steven recalled. "I felt like such a fool to have wasted precious time on such petty fights."

Steven found himself growing more and more resentful toward Patricia for dying. Even though he knew she did not want to die, he felt she was deserting him and the girls.

"I became depressed as I tried to deal with the bitterness that was growing inside of me. I was bitter with the faith healers, at people telling me God would not put more on me than I could bear, and I was bitter because He did not step in and heal Patricia the way I thought she should be healed," Steven finally revealed.

Bitterness spread rapidly through Steven, just as cancer had aggressively spread through Patricia. With the bitterness out of control Steven developed physical symptoms of exhaustion, headaches, nausea, and weakness. He began to worry he too would die; sleep eluded him.

"I had been around death so long, I thought I was also going to die. Then I worried about the girls. Who would take care of them? I had what seemed like superhuman strength when Patricia was ill. I went on very little sleep. But suddenly I found myself sick and weak."

During this time, Elizabeth, Steven's oldest daughter who was five, started bleeding from the rectum.

"I knew Elizabeth had cancer, too. I became more resentful toward God for what I saw as Him turning a deaf ear to my prayers. I just could not go through that ordeal, that agony, that horror again," Steven cried. "Who could bear going through cancer and death a second time with a loved one? Especially a child? How could I survive the death of my child? It was just too much. It was more than I could deal with."

After a couple of days in the hospital, doctors told Steven all the tests were normal and that Elizabeth had probably strained too hard when she had a bowel movement and that was the cause of the rectal bleeding.

Child care seemed to be too much of a demand on Steven. The girls took so much time, that Steven did not have time for personal needs. He resented being put in this position as a single dad and caregiver. The bitterness was growing out of control and Steven found that his health was declining more and more each day. As his health declined, his resentment grew and he stopped trusting in God. He stopped talking to God. He stopped praying.

Depression became worse when Steven tried to deny the negative feelings of anger, bitterness, and resentment that were growing inside. He kept telling himself that he should not have these feelings, what kind of a person would have such thoughts? Deep down he felt ashamed, embarrassed, and guilty over thinking such thoughts.

"I thought I was pretty sorry for feeling so bitter and angry. The fear was eating away at me. I was so afraid that I could not rear two girls alone. Then I felt guilty because of the bitterness and fear that were gnawing away at me. It was a vicious cycle," Steven said.

"My life was out of control. I was thrown into a lifestyle I had not chosen. I worried about the negative feelings eating away inside of me. I wondered if I was losing my grip on reality. I felt so isolated and lost."

How did Steven overcome the fear, bitterness, and guilt that threatened to destroy him?

"When I thought I was going to die, I called my parents. They lived in another state, but they came for me and the girls. I was checked into the hospital in my hometown by my family doctor. He ran several tests on me and the only thing he found was a small hernia. The three-day stay also provided the rest I needed," Steven sighed.

When he returned home, a friend gave Steven an article to read. The article dealt with the effects that the death of a spouse has on the surviving family members.

Steven thought he was losing grip on reality when he thought he saw Patricia standing in the doorway of their home one day. "I panicked and thought I was losing my mind. There were times I thought I smelled her perfume. At times, I thought I heard her footsteps.

"After I read the article, I realized what I had experienced was normal. But I still did not know how to get the feelings out," Steven remembers. "Beyond the pining and the yearning pangs, which occurred with regularity, I learned that as many as one-third of all newly bereaved people have experiences in which they hear, see, smell, or otherwise feel the presence of their dead spouse under a variety of circumstances."

Steven decided to seek help. He talked with a psychologist. The psychologist suggested Steven write Patricia a letter telling her how he felt and then burn it.

"By writing Patricia a letter I was able to say all the things I wanted to say. I told her everything I had wanted to say to her during her illness, but didn't, and how I felt right before and after she died. After I wrote the letter, I set a match to it, I burned it. As the smoke drifted upward, I felt like a weight had been lifted from my shoulders. I finally got the negative feelings out of my system."

Steven learned personal time had to be planned. He also learned the girls would do fine without him around all the time. The occasional overnight stays at the babysitter were good for him and the girls.

"When I reached the point where I was able to pray again, I realized I was going to make it," Steven said as he smiled. "It was not easy and at times I wondered if I would be able to deal with child rearing. The demands are overwhelming and exhausting at times."

So many of us are guilt-ridden. Guilt is the emotion we feel when we do something wrong, causing us to expect to be punished. Early philosophers referred to guilt as a judgment resulting from a violation of a moral law or common law. Sometimes our guilt is justified. Many times it is not. Our remorse may be of a mild form, stabbing us occasionally and causing discomfort. Or, we may let our unjustified guilt get out of hand, immobilizing us.

Jesus understood this. He healed many who were paralyzed. They felt hopeless and helpless by guilty feelings that had gotten out of control. The regret became so prominent in their minds that soon their body became incapacitated.

Are we better informed than our forefathers? Maybe so, but we are not any better at handling guilt than they were.

We are aware of the Almighty's love and what Jesus taught us about love. But somewhere along the way we have forgotten that self-love is not wrong. Selfishness is an emotion that can isolate us.

Self-centeredness is a distortion and perversion of love. Self-hate is pride's inseparable companion.

There are many types of guilt, but there are two categories of guilt that I want to address: leftover guilt and self-imposed guilt. Leftover guilt is learned from parental conditioning. Our family shapes our emotional patterns and ways of thinking by teaching us about feelings and what is the expected behavior within our family guidelines. We grow up hearing that we should not have done this or that, and we are made to feel guilty about our actions. We are made to feel guilty over things that really do not matter. Family uses guilt often times to manipulate each other into getting their own way in a situation.

Then, there is self-imposed guilt. Self-imposed is the feeling we have when we have broken a rule or moral code. Shame is the red flag that tells us when we have 'gone too far' and have crossed the line of acceptable behavior. Self-imposed guilt is the internal compass we use to gauge our behavior.

People who feel guilty will often avoid eye contact, they will fidget, or sit motionless, often they will stare off into space, shuffle their feet, or blush. They may become preoccupied with feelings of shame and have tunnel vision narrowing their perception of the world around them. They feel disconnected to what is going on around them.

Self-reproach can cause obsessive thoughts, resulting in compulsive acts trying to cancel out the obsessive thoughts. All-Consuming thoughts are intrusive and unwanted. There is a struggle to escape from these intrusions that are dominating our attention. These neurotic thoughts become trapped in an eternal loop that we can't escape from. A high degree of punctuality and rigid adherence to rules, strict orderliness, and perfectionism can be seen in the person's actions to try to relieve the stress of self-condemning thoughts. This obsessiveness is heartbreaking as we watch the person struggling to free themselves from this bondage.

Guilt leads to self-incrimination. Self-incrimination becomes an inverted form of good works, of inner penance which we feel we must do, thinking we are pleasing God. We hold a membership in an elite holy club which prides itself for self-belittling and putting guilt in our path as an obstacle to keep us in a constant state of shame. Somehow condemnation of self becomes the basis of "a good conscience." If we did not feel guilty; we would go to pieces from spiritual anxiety. We translate "Love your neighbor as you love yourself" into "Love your neighbor instead of yourself." This type of self-condemnation is not pleasing to God. It is harmful to those of us who carry it around. It becomes a burden that will literally weight us down.

We have to assess our personal philosophy, our spiritual and religious beliefs. If our guilt is left unchecked and allowed to grow, we soon find ourselves paralyzed. This crippling, self-imposed sinfulness can cause us to function on a slightly lower level or it may cause us not to function at all. In either case, we are not living up to our full potential. Unresolved condemnation can lead to alcohol abuse or drug abuse. Preoccupation with self-reproach may trap one into being unwilling and inflexible about learning coping skills. We feel that we do not have a choice about the situation and that past transgressions cannot be changed. We have literally trapped ourselves into a living hell on Earth.

It was once said that most of the patients in mental hospitals were not there because they were crazy, but because they are possessed by demons of guilt. There is a lot of truth to this statement. The psychological effects can include feelings of worthlessness or inferiority. Oversensitivity becomes a problem, as we begin to be obsessed with every aspect of right and wrong in the process of making any decision. Sometimes, we are not able to make a decision at all. This indecision will compound the problem of guilt, by making us feel even more guilt because of our inability to move forward in life.

So, how do we keep unjustified guilt from consuming us? We have to see that justified disgrace is healthy. When we have wronged another, this dishonor helps motivate us to set things right again. This is how it should be.

Needless regret, however, becomes a killer if we do not deal with it. When we are filled with misdirected misconduct, we imagine all kinds of unjust self-condemnation. People who are drowning in regret take complete responsibility for their mistakes. But they do not take into consideration any other factors that contributed to the problem.

What are some of the mental and emotional responses to grief?

- ~ Confusion/Disorientation—One may find it harder to complete an everyday task. And it may take one much longer to complete the same task that usually took only a few minutes to do.
- ~ Forgetfulness—In your grief, you may find it harder to concentrate on any activity. You may start a project and forget what you are doing while working on the task. It is as if your mind suddenly fell off a cliff.
- ~ Anxiety—Try not to become frustrated with yourself during this time of mourning. Get some extra rest and do not try to take on too many projects at a time.

~ Agitation/frustration—You may find that you have little patience with people, especially if they are complaining about trivial things. Frustration rears its ugly head and can set into motion a regretted respond to a minor inconvenience. You may find that overreaction to situations happens more often during this time in your life.

~ Concentration/lack of focus—During the grieving process, you may find that it is difficult to focus on what is going on around you. You may have problems being motivated. It may be difficult to even get out of bed in the mornings. You may have very little interest in completing tasks. Most activities may seem pointless and a waste of time.

~ Emotional numbness/shock—Especially during the first few months after a loved one's death, you may feel like you are just going through the motions of living. You may feel like you are walking around in a dazed fog.

The Almighty Father does not place unjustified sin in our minds. We do. He told us to love ourselves. We cannot love Him if we do not love ourselves.

We must realize that if worthless shame goes unchecked we are setting ourselves up for health problems. We must face unjustified guilt and ask Father to help us overcome this self-condemnation. We will have to turn our membership card from the elite self-condemnation club over to our Heavenly Father.

By turning our self-condemnation card over to Creator Source, we are asking not only for a peace of mind, but for help. We will need His help in overcoming guilt since we have a tendency to backslide.

There are a few things we need to remember as we overcome unjustified guilt.

1. We are not alone in our fight against unjustified guilt.
2. We are worthwhile.

3. We are lovable.
4. God loves us.
5. The superego can be harsh, punitive, and blaming. It can be self-destructive and damning toward us. We have to recognize the tactics of the superego and reject its self-destructive nature.

The most common results of guilt are anxiety, bitterness, and depression. We choose to either accept guilt or deny it. If we accept regret, we choose to continue to live in the past. If we do not face it head-on and deal with it, we continue to have bouts of anxiety and depression.

Unresolved remorse inhibits our thinking clearly, we are not able to enjoy life, and we become resentful. We may experience headache, stomachache, insomnia, mind-fog, irritation, depression, or anger among other physical and emotional symptoms. The fear of punishment for disobeying the scriptural teachings by a vengeful God is emphasized in many religions. We may develop health issues or a cancer or other life-threatening illness as a result of unresolved shame.

Here are some of the effects of unreasonable guilt:

~ Remorse can greatly affect our self-esteem. We feel worthless, hopeless, and unlovable.
~ It can weigh us down, preventing us from moving forward in life. We become stuck and feel like the weight of the world is on our shoulders. This can contribute to neck and shoulder pain. Lower back pain can manifest causing difficulty in completing daily activities. It can also contribute to our feet feeling heavy; legs and ankles swelling causing pain in our legs and difficulty in walking.
~ The emotional burden can literally make us feel "heavy" and result in physical weight problems. Or the burden can cause depression making us feel like we just can't move. We

have no energy. We are unable to get out of bed at times. We feel we are in a deep hole and can't get out. A lifeline or hand to grasp is needed to help pull us out of this hole.

~ It can lead to continuous self-criticism and problems with perfectionism. People who are perfectionists tend to suffer from anxiety, depression, and are more likely to commit suicide. A perfectionist is also more likely to have chronic or unexplained fatigue and pain syndromes like fibromyalgia.

~ Those who bear emotions of regret can become very apologetic, often saying, "I'm sorry" for even the most nonessential things. One problem that comes with low self-esteem is letting other people manipulate you and use you. The biggest problem or illusion with low self-esteem is that you will never know your true self-worth. Fear of making a mistake prevents one from living a full life, holding them back. The illusion of fear makes us feel as though our feet are stuck in cement and we are not able to free ourselves to move forward. A feeling of being permanently grounded in one place and not being able to free ourselves is despairing.

~ We can become paranoid about what others think of us, due to our own feelings of inadequacy. People experiencing paranoia believe that others are persecuting them. They may mistrust others and remain often in a constant state of suspicion. They are always looking over their shoulder, expecting the worst to happen.

~ Ongoing negative thoughts and emotions create changes within our physical body which can affect our physical health and lead to dis-ease. We may experience headache, stomachache, or numerous other symptoms. (1)

Guilt is not a nice feeling. It hurts. It feels prickly and uncomfortable, sticking its thorns deeper into our conscious mind. We try to avoid it as much as possible. We want to believe that we are not as bad of a person as we feel we are. We know that we have not lived up to our own standards of moral values making the stabbing pain worse. And when this happens, we find that we are spiraling down into a free fall that will be hard to pull out of. We see reality rapidly approaching us as we quickly plunge into this deception of guilt without a parachute to break our rapid descent.

Our emotional health depends on how well we cope with wrongdoing. The intensely painful feeling of guilt can make us experience erroneous feelings of believing that we are flawed and unworthy of love. Something we have experienced, done, or failed to do makes us feel unworthy of connecting to those we love and respect.

Having unresolved guilt can have an extremely detrimental effect because it can keep us from thinking clearly. We find it difficult to concentrate on the task at hand. Disgrace sucks the joy out of life making us feel drained and numb. Unresolved guilt can lead to bashing one's head on the wall of emotions, making us do penance of self-punishment. Resentment takes hold causing more pain than we can bear at times. Culpability is a feeling of responsibility or remorse for some offense, crime, or wrong, whether it is real or imagined. We are trapped in this emotional maze of mental pain. We cannot find our way out of the maze of emotions and we stay hopelessly lost in despair.

In addition to emotional pain, remorse can cause physical pain in the form of headaches, insomnia, and nausea. Condemnation is a powerful emotion that reminds us of the consequences of negative actions. It can also affect our future behavior. The stabbing pain from self-imposed shame can be pervasive enough to affect a person's well-being to the point of being debilitating.

Often times, some people experience difficulty when attempting to move past irrational guilt. This difficulty can lead to the development of chronic emotional issues such as depression and anxiety. Guilt and shame can be major motivating factors in other emotional problems like obsessive compulsive disorder. However, severe guilt can also make it difficult for an individual to sustain a relationship whether personal or social.

Shame is guilt's sibling causing painful feelings to arise from the depths of consciousness bringing up thoughts of something dishonorable or improper that is done by oneself or another person.

Shame must be resolved or our psyche will devise a plan to protect itself. We cannot continue to carry self-condemnation around for a prolonged period of time and survive physically or emotionally or spiritually. Harboring prolonged guilt takes its toll on us physically by showing up as disease. Our immune system becomes depleted and we are left defenseless. As an individual, we are not able to protect our body from prolonged condemnation, and our mind might turn remorse into bitterness. Our emotions will try to protect our physical well-being. They cannot know that by turning sinfulness into bitterness the problem is not resolved but compounded. Resentment breeds bitterness and instead of one emotional problem to deal with, we now have two.

Guilt, bitterness, and anger. The problem continues to grow. The roots tunnel deep becoming anchored deeper in the mind disorienting our thinking.

What can happen when bitterness tunnels deep within our mind? Can bitterness lead to anger? What can happen when anger gets out of control?

There are two sides to each emotion. There is the "light shining within" side that makes us feel good, that lets us know that we are contributing something worthwhile to ourselves and to society; and then there is the "shadow side" of each emotion. This is the dark side of the emotion that has become distorted and out of balance. This is the side of our psyche that we really do not want to admit that we have, not even to ourselves. It scares us to see this malevolence lurking within the shadows of our mind. Guilt is often thought of as a negative emotion. However, regret can prod us to right a wrong that we committed.

Unresolved and unchecked guilt is distracting and demoralizing. It affects our cognitive function causing us to have difficulty in focusing on the task at hand.

Other effects of regretfulness are:

~ it can destroy your self-esteem causing feelings of worthlessness, causing self-neglect and illness;
~ your self-confidence is likely to be diminished causing paranoia;
~ it can cause you to become your own worst critic causing loss of self-respect;
~ it can distort your perception of self and create self-doubt and fearfulness; and
~ it causes irrational thoughts about one's self and others.

Extended side effects on one's health from unfounded guilt can include increased irritability, bitterness, inability to show or experience joy, digestive symptoms including stomach upsets, increased blood pressure, chest pain, fatigue, headaches, and muscle pains to name a few complications.

By correcting our actions of wrongdoing, we have restored balance to the situation and to our life. Unfounded shame is a perversion to our emotional and physical health. We need to keep our perspective on this thought. Unfounded sin is unhealthy self-indulgence that keeps us separated from Source and keeps us in the dark abyss of depression.

What are we resisting when we do not or will not let go of guilt? How do we find the healing that we so desperately seek? What is the tool we need to use?

Acknowledge the action behind your feelings of regret. Is the guilt justified? In Steven's case, the self-condemnation was unjustified. Once the guilt is removed, what should we put into the space where culpability existed?

Once we realize the lie we have been telling ourselves about unjustified condemnation, we are able to put this emotion in the past. It becomes a lie, when the situation has been acknowledged and dealt with, if we keep revisiting the event. What truth do we put in that empty space?

We have to show ourselves compassion and lovingkindness. Well, how do we do this? Each time unacceptable guilt starts to creep back into our life, we need to stop and acknowledge the emotion we are feeling. At this point, we need to tell ourselves this is not justified and turn our attention to a more healthy thought process. Remember, that Source loves us unconditionally. If He loves us unconditionally, why are we refusing to show compassion to ourselves? Is God showing us unjustified compassion? If we feel God's compassion is unjustified, are we saying that Creator Source doesn't know what He's doing? How do we get out of this self-paralyzing cycle?

Once you realize that you have started back in the unjustified cycle of remorse, recognize it for what it is and stop it. Replace the emotion of regret with compassion and lovingkindness. Stop what you are doing and focus on becoming centered within your mind. Take a few deep breaths and let them out slowly. Bring your attention back to the reality that you are loved unconditionally, that you deserve this love that Father Almighty is offering to you. Receive this unconditional love with gratitude and thanksgiving.

Take a moment to tell yourself ten positive things about yourself. If you can't think of ten positive things about yourself, do not become stressed over this exercise. As time goes by, you will learn to love yourself as God the Father loves you.

What are some of the areas where you can love yourself? What affirmations can you tell yourself to engrain these truths into your heart? How can you free yourself from this vicious loop of lies you have told yourself?

Let's take a look at a few areas:

1. Father created you in His image. He loves you.
2. You have strengths just as everyone has strengths. Some strengths that you have could be: you are kind, you are loving, you are an asset to your family, friends, and job.
3. You are called to God and you are a member of His family.
4. You have truths to teach to others and help them realize their self worth.
5. You have the ability to share the love of I AM with others.
6. You have the ability to reach out to others to help them in a time of need.
7. You are created in the image of the Almighty and your Light of God shines from within you brightly, shining outward into the world.
8. You are a worthy child of All-That-There-Is.
9. You have the ability to help others see that they are a beloved child of Holy Spirit.
10. You have the ability to grow strong in the light and love of Universal goodness and love that Jehovah offers to everyone.

Self-forgiveness is the most compassionate thing you can do for yourself. When you forgive yourself you let go of that part of yourself, the part wanting to keep you trapped inside a continuous cycle of blame, shame, guilt, and fear. This way of living has you immobilized because you are dwelling in the past, trapped and stuck, preventing you from living in the present. Self-forgiveness is absolutely essential if you wish to become emotionally healthy and have peace of mind.

Pardon yourself from holding on to unreasoned guilt and let it go. Remember, stay in the present moment and when you notice that you are beating yourself up once again, practice letting go of the guilt, release yourself.

Why is it so difficult for us to move forward? Negative self-judgment and self-blaming can actually act as an obstacle to self-improvement. Self-forgiveness provides the opportunity to open the door to change. When you release resistance you are deepening your connection to yourself and to God.

Another obstacle to self-forgiveness is the desire to be seen and known as being a "good person." The image of being a good person was learned as a child. But, as often happens with children, we misunderstand the concept of being good and develop an unreasonable expectation of ourselves. Our "child" within often does not understand intellectual concepts of what a good person is or how to achieve that goal. Children are often concrete in thinking and cannot understand the subtle abstracts involved with emotions.

What steps do we need to take for self-forgiveness? How do you begin?

1. Self-understanding is essential. We have to understand what motivates us to hold on to unjustified guilt. Why do we wish to continue to punish ourselves?

2. By having compassion for yourself, for your own suffering, it can help you achieve the clarity needed to think of ways you can help yourself move past this nonrelinquished emotion.

3. Earn Your Own Forgiveness. Take responsibility, apologize, and make amends to yourself for sheltering false guilt.

4. Ask for forgiveness from your higher power, your God, your Creator.

Ask yourself, why do I insist on keeping myself held hostage over a situation that is unfounded? Write it down, look it over making sure that you have not left anything out. Then, like Steven, set a match to it and burn it, releasing it forever.

Dwelling on past mistakes does no one any good. Once you have an understanding on your motivations and why you insist on imprisoning yourself, unlock the doors of your prison cell and show compassion to yourself. If you are not able to show compassion to yourself, how can you possibly demonstrate compassion to others? Guilt affects our decisions and, in doing so, we often make the wrong decisions. Our decisions are not made on facts, but on judgmental external influence. Guilt is the one emotion that continues to manipulate us long past a reasonable period of time.

You must face the truth of the injustice that you have shown yourself. Whatever your religious or spiritual beliefs are, asking your higher power for comfort, compassion, and forgiveness can be a powerful step in forgiving yourself. This may be as simple as praying to your Creator to forgive you for your sins. A prayer as simple as, "I'm sorry. Help me to move past this self-imprisonment I have created," is enough to release you.

Another way to deal with guilt that you are erroneously nurturing is to just "let it go". You can make the decision in this very instant to let those feelings and memories just fade away. Imagine within your mind seeing it fading away like a rainbow after a rainstorm. Make a conscious decision to leave it behind and move forward. Refuse to spend any more time and energy on thinking about this judgement that you have placed on yourself. Stop punishing yourself! It serves no constructive purpose.

Why are you wasting energy on unfair guilt? Yes, I know, we are programmed to feel guilty. The programming starts as infants. It is inescapable, it is an overbearing cultural teaching that does not always motivate us to do better in life.

The truth is, guilt is the greatest destroyer of emotional energy. It leaves you feeling immobilized in the present by something that has already occurred. Guilt is a judgment that starts from internal influences. We take this internal influence and ingrain it into a perverted form of penitence. But, in doing so, we are making judgments on actions or thoughts that need no judgment. This judgment becomes an obstacle to our being authentic. This is a twisted thought process. By clearing away the illusion of guilt, this allows us to be more connected to what it is that we are experiencing. Our thoughts and our actions, in light of that experience, should help us to be more present with what we experience, with our emotions and with ourselves.

I AM has forgiven our sins and shortcomings. We have to forgive ourselves in accordance to His example. When we forgive ourselves, it becomes easier to forgive others. Harboring anger against ourselves is exhausting and it robs us from being the person God wants us to be. By not forgiving ourselves, we are being prideful. Forgiveness is a choice that takes courage, strength, and gives us the power to move forward. It gives us the opportunity to become an achiever rather than remaining a victim of our own self-condemnation.

We have lost contact with the divine spirit within us. We need to awaken the intrinsic consciousness within us. Pay attention to everything that surrounds you and be connected to the universal energy of life, the energy of God. Since the beginning of time, our thoughts, our emotions, our life choices have created the world we live in. The world in which we have set limits and boundaries for ourselves.

One of our greatest needs is to heal the emotions of loss, grief, and bereavement from the passing of a loved one. Any significant loss in a relationship or in our way of life can affect our health and we may feel like we are drowning in a sea of sorrow and desperation. This loss can create a deep valley of emptiness that we fear we can never overcome.

We have legions of angels standing by to lend us a hand, to pull us up to safety. Call on the Angel of Comfort to take your burdens and give to you the gift of acceptance and to guide you toward restoration of faith in the present and in the future. Prayer is our most powerful tool to use during this time of loss. The Angel of Comfort takes your tears and nourishes the seeds of hope, so that they will grow into fruits of light and renewal. The Angel of Comfort helps us see that we have the blessing of grace and helps us know that in our grieving, our loss has been acknowledged. Our loss has been recognized and honored.

While prayer is our most powerful tool, praying may be the hardest thing to do. We may feel that we are too wounded to pray. We may not even know how or what to pray. This can create another loss, the loss of connection with the Divine. Guilt from this suffering compounds the turmoil churning around within us. The Angel of Comfort will immediately connect us to the Divine Spirit within us. Comfort and compassion will be bestowed on us, giving us refuge.

Lift the veil between the subconscious mind and the conscious mind. Open the pathway to knowing that everything is a reflection of what we have created for ourselves.

The veil must be torn down between our subconscious mind and our conscious mind. Our subconscious mind is subject to holding onto every event we have encountered without understanding the meaning of what we experienced. Our conscious mind knows everything is a reflection of the creating self. Once you learn to align your conscious mind with your subconscious mind, you will see the absolute truth in everything. This altered state of consciousness moves you beyond your old programming, freeing you from the old wounds, transitioning you into a state of unlimited joy and happiness.

I AM gives us a feeling of permeant awareness.

PRAYER

I call on my guardian angel and the Angel of Comfort, to help me through these troubled waters. Please assist me in seeing this situation through new eyes. Inspire me to take a loving approach to the world around me and see the goodness that is there.

In this, my simple prayer, please release my sorrow and emptiness. Nourish my soul with your light of love. Turn my grief into courage so I can take the steps forward toward healing. Please turn this emptiness into feelings of gratitude for the time I had with my loved one. Help me honor their memory.

Help me reclaim the joy and pleasure that are still mine. I must remember that I am meant to live my life to the fullest in order to honor my loved one.

I know that the Angel of Comfort is with me during these times of loneliness and desparation, and will hold my hand and lift my soul up.

I ask for help in finding meaning in this time of crisis. Open my eyes to see the help that I can provide to others in need. I give thanks to my guardian angel and the Angel of Comfort for the blessings in this experience and reconnecting me to the love of God Almighty.

What happens when bitterness becomes uncontrollable? Can bitterness become a killer?

2

The Killer Within–
Bitterness

Danna felt bitterness toward her ex-husband Bill, and at times she felt pure unbridled hate toward him. Danna's bitterness also clouded her sunny disposition and unusually contagious smile. The darkness of her resentment toward Bill caused a shadow over her that hid her internal beauty that had shown outward. Bill had left Danna for another woman. This is the age-old story of the betrayal of a husband, seeking a younger woman and abandonment of his family. This, in itself, is ironic since Danna was only in her early thirties at the time of the betrayal. Although Danna had been a good wife and mother, she could not seem to get back on her feet after the divorce. Her anger had turned into raging bitterness. Her self-confidence had taken a hit and she found it hard to see that she is, indeed, an attractive woman who has so much to offer to others.

What Danna did not seem to realize was that bitterness and love cannot burn simultaneously in the same heart. Indulging in her animosity toward Bill began to affect her relationship with her children. Soon Danna's children were resentful toward her and they began to act out of control at times.

"I thought my children were going through a stage," Danna remembered. "I did not realize my asperity and resentment were causing my children to feel rejected."

By harboring an intense grudge and a burning resentment toward Bill, Danna was bound to let it spill over and injure her relationship with others, especially her children.

"I had been a good wife to Bill. I did not deserve to be discarded and thrown away. I had no idea anything was going on," Danna growled, "at least not then. Looking back I realize I did not want to see the signs that our marriage was in trouble."

The bitterness should have passed after the shock of divorce had time to wear off. Instead of moving ahead and starting a new life, Danna held onto her bitter anger, nurturing it and letting it grow like an ugly weed in a beautiful garden.

"I would not admit to myself that my vexation toward Bill was out of control at that point. I cultivated my hate, feeding it by reliving the events leading to the divorce and continued to nurture it. It grew into bitterness and formed a deeply grounded taproot in my mind. A taproot that became stronger and more deeply anchored as time slipped by. My self-indulgent behavior almost destroyed me. It almost destroyed my relationship with my children."

After fostering her hostility for several weeks, Danna begin to experience headaches. She became irritable and nothing pleased her. She wanted to sleep most of the time and had little energy or interest in caring for her children. Work of any kind was almost impossible for Danna to complete.

"When I first started having headaches I did not think much about it. Then they became more severe and I was having them more often. At this point I decided to see my family doctor. My doctor prescribed medication for the headaches. He called them tension headaches and told me to let him know if the medication was not helping," Danna said.

"Several more weeks passed and the headaches became more of a problem. By this time, I was so irritable the children began to avoid me altogether. I did not want to fix their meals or help them with their homework. I would come home after work and go straight to bed.

"I realized and I knew I had a real problem when I overheard my children one evening as they were talking to each other. Kelly, my daughter and the youngest, asked my son, Michael, 'Why doesn't Mama love us anymore?' I had to face the heart-breaking reality of my actions then and there. Kelly's words pierced my heart like a knife going through it, and I knew I had to get help," Danna recalls.

How did Danna overcome her bitterness and her hate toward Bill?

"I called my minister and made an appointment to see him," Danna explained. "When he told me my anger was sin and I should ask for forgiveness, I almost walked out of his office. I became enraged. He just was not telling me what I wanted to hear. I was the one who was betrayed by Bill. I was the injured one in this situation. I had every right to be angry."

Danna later learned that there were seven steps to go through in dealing with bitterness. Danna's minister used the basic steps Tim LaHaye taught in his book, *Understanding The Male Temperament*. (2) Danna's minister explained that she had to see her anger as sin. This was the *first step* and the hardest for Danna.

"I did not want to face my resentment. I did not want to face it as sin. It became sin when I held on to it and wanted revenge. I had indulged in self-pity for so long that the bitterness had become deeply entwined within me," Danna said.

The *second step* Danna had to take was also a learning experience.

"I had to learn to confess my angry thoughts or deeds when they occurred. By doing this, hatefulness could not become embedded again. I confessed often the first few weeks."

The *third step* Danna learned was to ask God to take away her angry pattern. This was not so easy since Danna was not really ready to give up her rage toward Bill. She had carried the fiery infernal rage within her for so long, that it was almost impossible for her to quench the blazing fire.

"My intense anger did not magically disappear when I asked God to take it away. I had to learn to give the problem over to our Creator," Danna admitted. "I kept taking it back. It took me a while to learn to let God take away the venom that had been spreading through me poisoning my soul. I had to let Father give me the antivenin to save my life from the deadly effects of this bitterness spreading throughout my being."

The *fourth step* was hard for Danna, also.

"I had to forgive Bill. It was very hard for me to forgive someone who had so willingly deceived me, hurt me, and made me so intently and bitterly angry. Bill had taken away my trust in the goodness of human nature. I could only forgive Bill when I realized my lingering bitterness would destroy me if I did not let go of it."

Step five perplexed Danna at first.

"I was to give thanks for anything 'bothering' me. I certainly could not understand why I should give thanks for the months of bitter pain I had felt. Then I understood that by giving thanks, I was trusting God to help me with this problem. By trusting Father to help me through this difficult time, I was also growing as a person," Danna said.

The *sixth step* made more sense to Danna and was easier for her to work toward.

"I was to think only of good, wholesome, and positive thoughts. Basically I am a happy person, but there were times . . . I remember thinking, 'It's been an awful day. Nothing good happened today.' But if I thought about the day, I could find something good about it. Some days I had to think harder than other days, but it worked," Danna smiled as she spoke.

"My cynicism did not disappear when I asked I AM to take it away. I had to learn to hand the problem over to my Comforter," Danna admitted. "I kept taking it back. It took me a while to learn to let Father God take away the bitterness and to allow Him to discard it."

The *seventh step* was the easiest to learn. Repeat the first six when you feel angry.

"I get mad about things at times and I am learning not to let the anger become bitterness again. It is easier to deal with anger when you first feel angry than it is when you let the roots take hold."

"Kelly sums it up in one sentence. 'Blow it off, Mama.' I think she's right," Danna says with a smile on her face. "At times it gets really tough, but with practice it gets easier to head off any embitterment before it gets started again."

Anger is a strong feeling of annoyance or displeasure or hostility. Anger is a warning that needs attention. If we ignore, mistrust, reject, and deny this warning device within us, our resentment can get out of control and become sinful. Are angry feelings best released in an explosive outburst or quietly suppressed? This debate continues in medical circles.

Blowing your top can be far more damaging than keeping your cool. People who are in the habit of "blowing their top" usually overexpress their anger and blow things out of proportion. This burning obsession results when the natural course of expressing anger is cut off and suppressed. Wrath is when a fiery emotion that is a wildfire burning out of control is physically experienced, and it requires a physical release. It is intended on destruction and the overwhelming need is its own immediate release.

Aggression is a hostile, destructive behavior that only compounds the emotional response in a situation. When an individual is blocked from attaining a desired goal, frustration occurs. Once this happens, the sense of frustration and the ensuing aggression increases to a point of a volcanic explosion. When this happens, there are three likely outcomes: conforming, or rebelling, or malevolent behaviors. If one denies anger and develops a behavioral pattern based on pretense, one might smile and comply with the other person's demands. Or, the anger will emerge as being passive-aggressive. If one rebels they will display a willing act of open resistance by digging in their heels and refusing to move forward. The third course of action is one of developing a malevolent or evil disposition. Healthy anger provides the foundation for relationships, whereas rage destroys relationships.

Repressed anger can lead to health issues as well. By turning this outrage inward onto oneself, illness and self-inflicted pain will began to boil to the point of overflowing into physical and psychological destruction. Research suggests that repressed anger contributes to gastrointestinal, respiratory, circulatory, headache, depression, and skin disorders.

What is the answer in dealing with anger? Is hatefulness in itself wrong?

Jesus became enraged with the money changers in the temple. He called them robbers and thieves. Tables were overturned and Jesus ran them out of the temple.

Exasperation in and of itself is not wrong. Anger becomes wrong when it is nurtured and held onto. Fury becomes wrong when it controls us instead of us controlling it.

The "cool reflective" approach is one way to deal with impatience. This approach is one that works in a balanced way. Both parties should calm down first, then discuss the conflict reasonably. If you can get at the problem, you can solve the conflict.

Expressing anger makes you angrier. It solidifies an embittered attitude and establishes a hostile habit. I once worked with a psychiatrist who would go into his office after seeing a patient and he would have a screaming fight. He would yell and knock things around in his office. This man developed kidney failure and subsequently died. I wonder if his outcome would have been different had he taken a different approach in dealing with frustration.

If you keep quiet during momentary irritations and distract yourself with pleasant thoughts or activity until you calm down, chances are that you will feel better and you will be better able to resolve the conflict. It is not enough just to express your irritation. You need to express your irritation in a calm manner that will enable communication to take place with genuine love and compassion between you and the other person. There has to be a genuine resolution of conflict or else the tension continues to build to a dangerous level.

A mild depression may occur in people who do not face their temper. Mild depression is found more often in women than in men. Some women may feel powerless and instead of getting mad, they get depressed. As a result, they may feel tired or have a chronic headachy feeling. They develop symptoms of overall pain in the muscles and nerve endings. They may develop a sense of helplessness and hopelessness and desperation.

Anger is a normal emotion. Expressing dissatisfaction is necessary for good health. The biggest problem we face is learning *how* to discharge it. The most successful way of dispelling annoyance is to understand the motive behind an aggressive action, then we can better deal with our feelings. The purpose of anger is to make a grievance known. If the grievance is not confronted, it will not matter if the frustration is kept in or let out.

There have been several studies that have connected anger to loneliness, chronic anxiety, depression, eating disorders, sleep disorders, obsessive-compulsive behavior, and phobias. Anger can also have a detrimental effect on our relationships and it threatens the development and preservation of our intimate interpersonal relationships.

Holding on to your grievance can cause you to have symptoms of:

~ elevated blood pressure,
~ increased heart rate,
~ tense muscles,
~ heart attack,
~ stroke,
~ hives,
~ asthma,
~ ulcers,
~ migraines,
~ low back pain or neck pain,
~ shortened life expectancy, and
~ brain fog,

After you have learned why you are irritated, give the provoker the benefit of the doubt. Try to come up with a reasonable justification for the behavior in this situation. It is never all one person's fault in a disagreement. It takes two to argue.

Take time out. Calm down and then discuss the conflict rationally. You may find it helpful to walk away from the situation until you have had time to calm down.

Making your grievance known without attacking the other person helps get your point across without adding fuel to the flames.

Listen to what is being said. Really listen closely. Give up on thinking about what you want to say next instead of hearing what the other person is telling you. By listening you can better understand what has just happened.

Forgive the other person for their part in the conflict. Then forgive yourself if needed. Forgiveness is necessary for one to be able to move forward. Forgiveness is not accepting or agreeing with what happened, but acknowledgment that it is time to move beyond the anger. It is letting go. It is releasing yourself from this debilitating grief.

Points to remember:

1. Releasing is an act of the will. It begins in your head, not in your emotions. It is a conscious decision.
2. Whenever angry thoughts emerge, you should stop them immediately and remind yourself that you are forgiving that person.
3. Showing mercy is a growth process, not an instantaneous experience. Remember, Father God shows you mercy every single day of your life. He expects us to do the same for those people we are in conflict with.
4. Eventually the heart catches up with the head and the release is complete. It becomes a dead memory.
5. Forgiveness is giving up your right to get even. (3)

We must take a look at our motives when we become exasperated with another person. Do we really desire and want to get even? Why? Do we retaliate? Does your hatred stem from an injured ego? Do we wish to take advantage of the other person? If so, this is negative energy and self-destructive. It must be confessed, released, and forgiven. We must accept the reality of our wrath toward the other person.

Anger should produce a loving confrontation instead of pouting, or gossiping, or ending the relationship. The air must be cleared, not only to repair the strained relationship, but also to prevent our imagination from running wild. Imagined injustice can lead to imagined fears. Fears of retaliation on the part of the other person, to get even with us can cause the fears to become paranoia or a phobia.

When you are annoyed, look at the details in the situation and you will find strong physical sensations of tightness, a tensing sensation, or burning sensation. Anger is a fiery emotion full of hot, burning, flaming destructive energy. If you do not want to be caught up in anger, bring your attention right into these physical sensations. Be mindful of the physical sensations you are feeling. By doing so, it will help to dissipate this stormy energy. (4)

Angered pain is not necessarily a problem, and it is not always under your control. What matters is how you relate to the disappointment once it has presented itself. If you dwell and linger over the stormy, energetic sensations and convince yourself that your thoughts are true and justified, rage overtakes you before you realize it. But there is an alternative: feel the sensations and tell the truth about the incident. Then anger becomes an ally revealing more deeply the essence within you. (4)

What are the effects when you are angry? Anger pushes people away, scares them, makes them fight back or shut down.

Remember that anger or any reaction is not the fault of the other person, you are responsible for your own reaction to the situation. If you are upset, look within yourself. Oftentimes, we see in ourselves qualities in the other person that we do not like in ourselves. Those qualities that we do not like in the other person are being mirrored back to us, reminding us that we too have the same disposition that has upset us. Investigate what has been triggered within you, and your whole perspective on the situation will shift. (4)

If we are holding on to inflamed feelings against someone who has wounded us, we can't be in a right relationship with God. His call is for us to forgive as He has forgiven us of our own sins. Do not wait to obey Father's call until you feel like forgiving because chances are you probably never will. We need to decide to forgive despite our feelings, and as we trust Jehovah to help us in the forgiveness process, our feelings will completely change along the way.

Once anger is purged from your system, consider filling this space with peace and calmness. Do whatever you can to bring in peaceful feelings and a sense of inner calmness. Take a walk in nature, visit with friends, listen to music that makes you happy, mediate, or pray, any of these activities can bring you into a place of reflective peacefulness.

But what happens if we do not purge the bitterness? How can it affect our health? What is the price we pay for nurturing bitterness?

The stress hormone cortisol is released during stressful moments and chronically high levels of cortisol can disrupt the immune system making one vulnerable to developing a number of diseases. It is important to find a new purpose in life to stop the detrimental destruction to your health, both physically, emotionally, mentally, and spiritually.

Do you really what to be known as a bitter person? Do you want to speak unkind words to the people who you love? Do you want to be hostile and use harsh words to those around you? If you do, you will find that you are isolated because of your behavior. Your criticism of and to others takes the focus away from your own shortcomings. We disrespect other people when we are bitter. Holding on to bitterness keeps you locked into the past. Is this the life you really what to live?

What happens when we forgive ourselves and others and let go of bitterness? Forgiveness means different things to different people. Generally, it involves a decision to let go of resentment and thoughts of revenge. Resentment and revenge require a tremendous amount of energy to maintain. This mind-set can and will exhaust you mentally and physically. It is a heavy burden to carry on your shoulders and it will break you and drop you to your knees if it is not relinquished.

Forgiveness leads to feelings of understanding, empathy, and compassion for ourselves and others. Forgiveness does not mean that you will necessarily forget or excuse the harm done to you. What it does mean is that you are ready to regain your peace of mind, your sense of balance and to move forward in life.

Forgiveness means that you are willingly bringing peace into your life. When you move away from suffering, you reap the fruits of your actions by choosing to move forward by forgiving yourself and anyone else involved in the situation. We learn to recognize the value in forgiveness and will see improvement in our life. Move away and out from the role of victim. In doing so, you release the control and power that bitterness has had over you. As you let go of grudges, you will no longer allow bitterness to define your purpose in life.

Some of our greatest and most frustrating pain comes from stresses in our relationships with people in our lives. The deepest pain can come from those whom we love dearly. Betrayals wound us deeply and we may feel that we can never forgive. We have to forgive before healing can begin. If we do not forgive, we will wither and die.

Dwelling on what has happened allows bitterness to become a permanent component of our character. It becomes an ugly tattoo that scars our character causing our self-image to erode from being a competent, self-assured, and a purpose-driven person to that of a helpless victim.

Do you want to stay trapped in the past? Really? Do you? Bitterness can make one so self-protective that you view the entire world through a cynical eye, avoiding opportunities and relationships that could be fulfilling for you. Do you want to live behind a wall of hate that you have imprisoned yourself behind? By dwelling on the past hurt, you are doing just that, living in the past. In reality, you are not living at all, because there is no life in the past. You are just going through the motions of living and missing out on the wonders of being in the present. By prolonging your pain, you are holding yourself back from moving forward in living and you are blinding yourself of the opportunity that is standing right in front of you.

People who are bitter usually spend a great deal of time replaying the event, retelling the story, and spinning it more and more out of control with "if only that had not happened" scenarios. This takes time and energy away from resources that are far more important than whatever has been taken from you.

Why do you continue to hold on to bitterness? In some cases, resentment becomes a sense of purpose for some people. Dissatisfaction becomes our banner for self-worth. We use it to justify our stance in the situation. It provides a scapegoat to hide from our fear of failing. This is also a way of avoiding responsibility for making our decisions and taking action to build the kind of life that we truly want to live.

Disgruntlement can drive away the people we love and suddenly we find we are alone with no one to love or who loves us. Clearly, bitterness not only destroys your life, but the life you had with those you do love. You become the stereotype of the lonely bitter old man or woman that is often portrayed in movies and literature.

Bitterness is a maze that can entrap us for a lifetime if we are not careful. It is easy to get lost in the hallways that lead to the dead-end of disappointment, anger, and fear. The indignation that one harbors toward another person and the emotional punishment that is embedded in your heart has precisely the opposite effect over time than what you think it will. Spitefulness does nothing to the person you are angry with, but it quietly and steadily destroys you. You are slowly being poisoned by your own hardheadedness and hardened heart. Resentment kills those who harbor it and hold on to it. By refusing to release this chronic pain, you have just signed your own death sentence.

Unhappiness grows out of control when we refuse to uproot the feelings of betrayal that are felt when someone has hurt us. We feel that they have taken something of importance away from us and that we can't get that sense of trust back. If we are not careful, hostility can make us do and say foolish things. We find that we are comfortable in wallowing in a cesspool of negative thinking, remembering every little detail of the betrayal to justify our emotional attitude of resentment and anger.

This only isolates us even more from having a meaningful and loving relationship with others. Funny thing is, our memories are flawed and the longer we hold on so tightly to the bitterness, the more distorted our thinking becomes in our mind. The situation has been blown up out of proportion compared to what really happened. However, this can lead to our emotional and spiritual suicide. One has to realize that you alone are responsible for what you think, feel, and say. No one else can make us bitter. Our emotions are just that, ours. This acrimonious emotion is a trap that we can find ourselves snared in if we are not careful. It is important to remember that we have to purge the negative feelings of bitterness and antagonism from our life if we want to survive.

When we call on the Angel of Forgiveness to help us release the bitterness and anger that we are feeling, we must remember that forgiveness is not a sign of weakness. It is a sign of deep inner strength. We are leaving the state of being a victim behind and building spiritual strength that allows for growth. Progress can be made toward becoming whole and in unity with God only as we learn to forgive.

As adverse thoughts and feelings begin to boil and bubble to the surface, we are able to release these negative feelings faster and prevent them from taking hold in our conscious minds again if we are willing to let go of this negative energy that is trying to escape from within us. We are able to prevent being drowned and carried away in a tsunami of emotional agony once we release the anger dwelling inside of us. The Angel of Forgiveness empowers us with love and blesses us by helping us move from these adverse feelings and helps us put them behind us.

We are taught in (Eph 4:32) "AND BE YE KIND ONE TO ANOTHER, TENDERHEARTED, FORGIVING ONE ANOTHER, EVEN AS GOD FOR CHRIST'S SAKE HATH FORGIVEN YOU."

Can you do that for yourself? Can you show yourself kindness and forgiveness? Hand the bitterness over to Father. Until you do, you will continue to have the sour taste of bitterness in your mouth. Clean the bitter aftertaste from your mouth with the cleansing freshness of forgiveness. Let go and hand this bitter plate of self-destruction over to your Savior. Do not wait! Do not delay! Do it right now! Hand it over to the one who will happily take this burden from you.

PRAYER

I call on the Angel of Forgiveness and my guardian angel, please assist me in seeing this situation through new and compassionate eyes. Help me to see this event through eyes of lovingkindness and empathy.

I remember the situation that created this stabbing, sorrowful pain and the person who I place this blame on for this tragic situation. I release the binding bitterness that I have held this person imprisoned in for so long. I open the cell door of this prison that I have kept not only this person in, but also myself as well. I choose to release us both from this imprisonment of pain. I ask the Angel of Forgiveness to help me transform this hurtfulness of immobility and sadness into joy and to fill my soul with the compassion that Father God shows to me by helping me in forgiving the person who has hurt me.

I give praise to I AM THAT I AM, ALL-THAT-THERE-IS for helping me to see the Truth in this situation and for assisting me in releasing the lingering pain from this festering wound that I have been carrying in my heart. I am grateful for this lesson in forgiveness and ask the Angel of Forgiveness to move me in the direction of teaching others how to forgive as I have learned how to forgive. AMEN.

Guilt, bitterness, fear. The problems continue to build. What happens when fear, whether real or imagined, becomes a phobia?

3

The Gripping Bonds of Fear

"When I was being held at gunpoint, I was not afraid until I got home. Then it hit me. It hit me real hard; when I realized how close I had come to death. I look back on the situation and I still can't believe that it happened to me," Ann says as she shutters.

"I never thought I would be looking down the barrel of a snub-nosed gun. Somehow I kept my wits throughout the two-hour ordeal. But later that night, when the fear began to take over, I could not keep a grip on myself, my emotions began to run wild.

"My heart began to race again. My breathing became short and fast. My legs became weak and I was trembling. Perspiration broke out over my entire body and my mouth was so dry I could hardly speak. The knot in the pit of my stomach became so tight, I thought I would get sick and vomit."

Terror signals us to stop, look, listen, and then act in a way that will protect us. Horror becomes a problem when we are unable to cope with it. When this happens, we direct most of our actions toward escaping this paralyzing fear.

Being a young, energetic woman, Ann was shocked to find herself in a life-threatening situation.

"When I met Jim, I was trying to pick up the pieces of my life. I had just gone through a divorce and was working full-time as a nurse in a local hospital and then later on in a physician's office. I needed a friend and Jim made me laugh. He seemed to know just about everyone I knew and no one warned me about him," Ann recalls.

As the weeks turned into months, Ann realized Jim had serious mental health issues. She wanted to help him.

"Jim had low self-esteem, but he knew how to use it to manipulate people. He told me about the death of his mother and about problems he had in a previous marriage. He seemed to be searching for a relationship with God."

Ann tried to share her faith with Jim. She wanted Jim to know the love and comfort Christ could give to those who hurt.

"About a year after I met Jim, I began to realize he was trying to control my life. He would get mad when I went out on dates. I finally saw that I had to give up the relationship with Jim and move on.

"That was a difficult decision for me. I'm not one to give up. But I should have broken off the friendship months earlier. My hard-headedness just would not let me. I should have listened to my inner voice warning me and walked away right then and there.

"I went to Jim's apartment to return a record album that he had loaned me from his collection of old vinyl records. I asked him to stay away from me, it was then that he pulled a gun on me," Ann shuttered as she recalled the incident.

Having worked with psychiatric patients, Ann relied on her nursing experience to get control of the situation.

"Jim had lost control. It was like he was being possessed by some unknown power. I could tell by the dark look in his eyes something evil was in control," Ann said as she tried to control her emotions. "Jim threatened suicide, but I had no doubt in my mind that he would shoot me, not himself if I turned around to walk away."

After Ann got Jim to put the gun down, she left. Ann called the family physician she was working for when she got home.

"I needed to be reassured that I had done the right thing. I also wanted him to call Jim and get Jim to see a psychologist," Ann said.

Thinking the worst was over, Ann tried to put the incident behind her. Then about a month later, Ann experienced her first phobic reaction as she was going home from work.

"The attack was so sudden and it came out of nowhere. The speed at which it developed was lightning fast. It dominated my mind and emotions. I was reliving the experience all over again," Ann remembers.

The irrational dread and panic in a harmless situation baffled Ann. When she started to develop the physical symptoms she experienced the day Jim pulled the gun, Ann knew she had to do something.

"I knew if I did not get control of myself that this phobic reaction would become serious. I had to confront the situation head on."

How did Ann work through her fear?

"I knew not to try to deny my feelings," Ann said, recalling the steps she went through. "I had to accept the fact that the fear would return. I knew I could not try to ignore the fear when it did return. If I tried to block it, things would only get worse for me."

By accepting the fact that the nightmare would return, Ann was confronting what she felt.

"When the fear did return a week or so later, I waited. I let it be."

Waiting helped Ann get control of her feelings. She told herself that it would get better.

"While I was feeling the panic, I continued with my work. I talked with my patients and answered the phone. I dealt with what was instead of what if."

Monitoring her uneasiness helped Ann keep a grip on her emotions.

"I learned how to function while I felt the anxiety. This helped the phobic reaction diminish."

Knowing that the fear could reappear helped Ann realize that if it did, it was not a relapse. If the phobic reaction did recur it should be used as an opportunity. By regarding the opportunity to study why it happened helps diminish the problem even more. Examine how you are going to handle the crisis. Make sure every effort is being used to practice placing attention on the phobia.

"I was lucky," Ann says, "I had a mild reaction. I know people who have had severe phobic reactions. Their fright has held them in captivity and refused to allow them to live a normal life. It is a problem that happens to a lot of people. I now have a better understanding of what they are going through."

"I will not be so quick to say, 'That's silly to let fear control you.' It comes on suddenly and before you know it, **bam**, distressful panic has gripped you. But there is hope for those dealing with a phobic reaction."

Yes, the gripping bond of this turbulence can be broken. And with time, patience, practice, and help, you can be shouting, "I'm free at last!"

When we are consumed with overwhelming apprehension we lose control over our perception of what is occurring. A phobia is an irrational, involuntary, and inappropriate reaction to the situation. If we can find a peace of mind in the midst of our distress, we can learn we do not have to be afraid. We learn how to be responsible for anything we experience and to our reaction within the situation.

Fear is a vital response to physical and emotional danger, and if we did not feel the threat, we could not protect ourselves from legitimate trepidation.

A definition of the psychology of fear would distinguish it as an emotion and also as a feeling. Fear can be conscious, or fear can be unconscious with bodily reactions, and dismay can be without bodily reactions. Also, alarm is found in anxiety and there is fear in phobias.

Fearfulness is closely related to, but should also be distinguished from, the emotion of anxiety. Anxiety occurs as the result of threats that are perceived to be uncontrollable or unavoidable. The fleeing fear response also serves as a survival response by generating appropriate behavioral reactions. So, this response to a fleeing fear has been preserved throughout evolution for mankind's longevity to continue. The "flight or fight" response is the great force that promotes our self-preservation.

There are many fears, but here are four common fears that people deal with:

~ There is the Invitational Fear that encourages us to meet a deadline at work or school. It keeps us motivated to take the next step to complete the task at hand. We feel the pressure as the deadline nears.

~ Then there is the fear of Trauma. Trauma fears are usually irrational and can flare up with the slightest occurrence, causing a fight, flight, or freeze reaction that no one who's witnessing it can understand why it is happening.

~ The Warning Fear is associated with the "flight or fight" response to a dangerous situation. This is a legitimate fear that shows up to tell us to take a course of action that is correct and necessary in order to avoid injury or serious harm.

~ The last common fear is that of the Ego. In this type of fear, it can be irrational causing us to protect ourselves in situations that may not be harmful at all. This fear tells us to protect ourselves from people who do not look like us or who do not share our core belief systems. It prevents us from experiencing the differences between people and cultures.

Other types of apprehension are:

~ pain—most of us want to avoid physical and emotional pain, especially extreme pain that can be detrimental. While pain has a purpose in making us attend to an injured body part, we still struggle with the sensations of pain when it continues after we have addressed the issues with the injured body part. Psychological pain is just as painful as physical pain and has to be addressed so one can find relief.

~ loss—we find that we have attachments to people and things. Fear of losing something or someone is a strong motivator. We fear the loss of a job, which, in turn, grows to the loss of our home, or our car and other possessions we have acquired. Our most intense fear with loss is the loss of someone we love whether it is through death or abandonment.

~ nongain—we are fearful that we will not have the money we need to survive or the money we want to gain a higher level of status. The thought of not gaining the things and status we desire can produce anxiety and fear about not only the present, but also with our future.

~ death—death frightens most of us. The fear of the unknown and what happens after death is terrifying to many of us. Often, people seek condolences in religion or a higher power.

~ uncertainty—we can't predict the future and we can't always predict the outcome in a certain situation. We want to "know" what will happen at any given time, at each step of life. Are we going to be able to reach our goals? Are we going to be under the control of someone else and not in control of our own destiny?

~ failure—we often do not try new things because of the fear of failure. Missed opportunities slip through our fingers because we are worried we will look foolish if we fail.

~ fear—humans have a tendency to fear just about anything and everything.

Franklin D. Roosevelt's famous speech, "Only Thing We Have to Fear Is Fear Itself," pretty much summons it up in this one sentence.

We have to look beyond the illusion of fear. Fear is the energy that contracts and destroys you, while love is the energy that develops and builds you.

A phobia is an extreme, irrational fear of a specific object or situation. Phobias are thought to be a learned emotional response. It is generally thought of as phobias occurring when fear is produced by an original threatening situation that is transferred to other similar situations. Often the original fear has been repressed or forgotten.

Panic disorder strikes between three and six million Americans, and is twice as common in women as in men. It can appear at any age. It is also noted that, in the U.S. and Europe, approximately one-half of the individuals with panic disorder have expected panic attacks as well as unexpected panic attacks. Panic attacks are often accompanied by other conditions such as depression or alcohol and drug use to try to cope with or prevent the symptoms associated with fearfulness. Phobias can develop, causing symptoms to develop in places or situations where panic attacks have occurred in the past.

Can you have a panic attack when you are sleeping? Yes, these freezing, motionless attacks can happen, waking you up from your sleep with no obvious cause. You wake up with having difficulty breathing, you are drenched in sweat, you are confused and disoriented. People who have nighttime panic attacks may find it difficult to calm down and go back to sleep. When nocturnal panic attacks happen, they can disturb the sleep of your partner and make it difficult to stay awake during the day. Studies have suggested that between 50 to 70 percent of people with panic disorder will experience at least one panic attack at night.

What should you do if you are awaken during the night with a choking panic attack? Get up out of the bed and become fully awake so you can work through the episode. Accept that the attack happened and observe the feelings that have surfaced. Be in the moment and breath through the fear. Deep breathing will help reduce the stress that the attack has caused and help you to calm down. If you find that you are not able to relax enough to go back to sleep, engage in a boring task that you do not normally like to do such as folding the laundry or cleaning the kitchen.

Practice good sleep hygiene.

1. Establish a presleep routine. Shower or bathe in warm water before bedtime. Have the bedroom temperature a little cool to promote comfort while you sleep. Bedrooms are for sleeping and sex. Keep the TV and electronics out of the bedroom as much as possible. Have a comfortable mattress. Turn off the lights and if you must have an alarm clock turn it to where you are not looking at the display screen. Pets often disturb one's sleep. You may want to either make sure your pet has its own bed or find another room for your pet to sleep.

2. Do not watch the news just before going to bed. People often get caught up in the "worrying about world events" and find it hard to calm their mind before sleep.

3. Go to bed at the same time every night and get up at the same time every morning. If you find that you are not

able to go to sleep within ten to fifteen minutes of going to bed, get up until you feel like you are getting sleepy.

4. Do not take a nap during the day. Daytime naps interfere with the sleep cycle causing us to be wakeful at night.

5. Limit caffeine during the day and restrict its use in the afternoon and evening hours. Also cigarettes and some over-the-counter medications can cause sleep disturbances. Studies show that warm milk will help induce sleep. Milk contains an amino acid called L-Tryptophan which helps the body to produce melatonin and serotonin. These two chemicals activate the body to induce sleep. By drinking milk before bedtime, you can cause your body to produce these chemicals, causing you to start to feel drowsy.

Anxious people can have interference with realistic thinking which is readily observed. A vicious cycle of escalation in unrealistic thinking can occur causing more anxiety. Highly anxious people experience difficulty in learning new complex and difficult assignments.

These observations can include:

~ repetitive thinking about the danger;
~ reduction in the ability to reason and evaluate and reappraise objectively one's thoughts;
~ overreaction both psychologically and emotionally to stimuli that are viewed as dangerous;
~ difficulty with short-term memory and loss of words when speaking or writing;
~ difficulty in concentrating on immediate tasks;
~ hypervigilence to surroundings; and
~ the tendency to dwell on negative outcomes in different situations;

The physical manifestations of panic and anxiety attacks include:

~ sweating profusely,
~ shaking uncontrollably,
~ muscle contractions,
~ insomnia,
~ feeling exhausted,
~ difficulty breathing,
~ nausea,
~ increased heart rate,
~ chest pain,
~ hypertension,
~ dry mouth and trouble swallowing; and
~ feeling that you are going to die,

What are some of the causes that can play a role with panic attacks? While research continues to investigate causes other than environmental factors, these are some of the known causes:

~ genetics
~ adaptive changes in brain function resulting from other medical or psychiatric conditions
~ overstimulation by thoughts or by environmental cues
~ expectations that are incompatible with abilities
~ inability to act

How do we find peace of mind? How do we learn to be responsible for what we experience? Can we be cured of our phobia?

A deeply ingrained irrational fear can be changed by shifting our focus. We have to shift our focus away from the fear of past preconceptions, or future unknowns. A panic attack takes a very powerful emotional toll on the person affected.

Be in the moment, stay focused on what is going on in this current point of time. By shifting our focus to the present and using the time to become centered, we will begin to find peace. Remember that panic attacks are self-limiting and usually last about ten minutes.

Worry, guilt, and fear are all emotions that drain us of our vital energy and strength. This limiting and restricting energy could be used to nourish and heal us instead of letting it deplete our strength. A steady diet of anger, fear, and resentment can have devastating consequences on our health.

Living under a constant threat weakens our immune system. It can cause cardiovascular damage, you may experience gastrointestinal problems such as ulcers or irritable bowel syndrome, and it can cause decreased fertility and impetus in both men and women. Worry can impair short-term memory and interfere with the formation of long-term memories. Chronic fear can cause damage to certain parts of the brain, such as the hippocampus. Irrational fear can impact our relationships with others and prevent us from developing deep and meaningful attachments with others. It robs us of being intimately connected to another person.

Many of us have believed that the past predicts the future. In reality, the past has no relevance in regard to our future. The present moment in time is what counts and is all that we really have. Once we learn to live in the present moment, and we learn that thinking of the future is an extension of that moment, then we have opened ourselves up to healing. We have to remember that the future is not carved in stone and that we have free will to shape our future as we see fit.

When fearful feelings take over ask: What's upsetting me? What is making me hold on to it? What do I really want?

Turn loose of the emotions. Imagine throwing them as far away from you as possible. Remember, our emotions are a conscious decision and we do have control over them.

There are many theories about what causes phobias. Often a phobic person knows exactly what triggered their problem: a physical illness, domestic stress, loss of a loved one, stress at work, a domineering parent or partner. Usually an abnormal fear starts with an inexplicable panic attack. If the attack occurs in a crowd, crowds become fearful reminders of it. Then the obsessive dread takes on a life of its own.

Practice is an essential part of recovery. Those who are best able to practice dealing with their fears on a daily basis are the ones who do the best. The more often you are able to confront the phobia and work through it, the intensity of the attack will begin to lessen in severity and duration.

We should try to view a panic attack as an opportunity to practice going through the fearful episode the right way until it no longer upsets us. By doing this, the exposure will help lessen the affect that the phobia has on us.

A more realistic goal is to teach ourselves how to lead a normal life by confronting, rather than avoiding, feared objects or situations. By confronting these situations we can begin to develop a positive attitude toward the alarm we feel. It is hard to find the courage to face these challenges at times, but often it is easier to find the courage you need to face the situation when you have a good support system in place. The challenge becomes a little less daunting when we have a trusted friend or family member with us as we face our phobia.

We can admit that our fears are irrational. But to insist there is a basis for an irrational fear is paranoia and not a phobic behavior.

Knowing our desperations are unfounded does not lessen the impact of the panic we are trying to deal with. Panic attacks are self-limiting. The usual frightening symptoms of a phobia are dizziness, lightheadedness, weak legs, difficulty in breathing, and fears of impending death or insanity.

Phobia therapists tend not to speak in terms of a cure for their patients. They emphasize to the patient that they learn to fear their fear less. By doing so the distress will diminish, although it may not disappear completely.

For those who have a more severe form of a phobia, it is comforting to know phobias are among the easiest to treat. A combination of group therapy, relaxation techniques, diet changes, family support, and gradual exposure to fear-provoking situations have been proven to be very good therapy.

When an impending anxiety attack happens, say to yourself, "Okay, phobia, fine, let's get it over with," and the panic attack will pass more quickly. It's when we try to fight the panic that it comes faster and hits harder. If we withdraw from our fears and try to distract ourselves, we are running away.

Accepting our panic attacks will help us overcome what is happening. Fighting brings more tension, more sensitization, and further illness. Remember telling someone not to think about a certain word or situation? What happens? That word or situation is all they can think about. This is the same principle in dealing with phobic attacks. The more you try not to deal with it when it arrives, the harder time you have in getting over it. Try walking against the wind. What happens? You exert more energy trying to walk against the wind. It becomes exhausting! Now, try walking with the wind to your back. What happens? You have the wind at your back helping you in your journey. You are not expending as much energy and you do not become worn-out from the experience. Anticipatory guidance provides the individual with both knowledge of a potentially stressful situation and techniques on how to cope with it.

Imagine yourself floating as if you are laying on a raft on a lake. Think, "relax and enjoy floating on the raft, do not fight it." Do deep breathing exercises during this moment. This will help you release enough tension to encourage movement. Then let time pass, have patience with yourself.

A phobic reaction binds its victim with two fears. First comes the fear of crowds or bridges or whatever the trigger event represents. Then comes the second fear, the fear of the first fear, the dread of losing control and doing something embarrassing or dangerous in public. The saying, "divide and conquer" is the best way to deal with these problems. Deal with each phobia, one at a time.

By imagining our worst fears, by deliberately seeing them in vivid detail we can view them in context. What is happening during this moment? Are you alone, or in a crowd? What is going on? What do you see, smell, feel, hear, taste? By doing this, we can alleviate much of our anxiety. When we alleviate our anxiety, we gain control over our fears. By gaining control over our fears, we find that we do have peace of mind.

Posttraumatic stress disorder (PTSD) is a mental health condition that's triggered by a terrifying event. The event was by either experiencing it or witnessing it. Symptoms may include flashbacks, nightmares, and severe anxiety, as well as uncontrollable thoughts about the event. (5)

Many people who go through traumatic events may have temporary difficulty adjusting and coping, but with time and good self-care, they usually get better. If the symptoms get worse, last for months or even years, and interfere with your day-to-day functioning, you may then have PTSD. (5)

PTSD symptoms are generally grouped into four types: intrusive memories, avoidance, negative changes in thinking and mood, and changes in physical and emotional reactions. Symptoms can vary over time or vary from person to person. (5)

PTSD is most notably seen with military personnel, but it is being recognized more often in civilian life. PTSD is recognized in children as well as adults.

Symptoms of negative changes in thinking and mood may include:

~ negative thoughts about yourself, other people, or the world;
~ hopelessness about the future;

~ memory problems, including not remembering important aspects of the traumatic event;
~ difficulty in maintaining close intimate relationships;
~ feeling detached from family and friends;
~ lack of interest in activities you once enjoyed;
~ difficulty experiencing positive emotions; and
~ feeling emotionally numbed; (5)

Symptoms of changes in physical and emotional reactions (also called arousal symptoms) may include:

~ being easily startled or frightened;
~ always being on guard for perceived danger;
~ self-destructive behavior, such as drinking too much or driving too fast;
~ trouble sleeping;
~ trouble concentrating;
~ irritability, angry outbursts, or aggressive behavior; and
~ overwhelming guilt or shame; (5)

There are four levels of defense against anxiety:

1. Changing the environment or your perspective
2. Character development through repetitive socially approved behaviors
3. This line of defense comprises the repressive defenses that fall into the categories of: keeping conflicting ideas out of one's awareness, those aimed at inhibiting attention, concentration, conscious awareness, memory, emotions, sensory stimulation, and motor and visceral functioning, defenses of displacement and phobic avoidance, undoing through compulsive rituals
4. Regressive defenses and involves a return to a state of helplessness, withdrawal from reality by means of

internalization of hostility with suicidal tendencies, and acting out of repressed sexual or hostile impulses

With PTSD, it's not as much about what the person experienced or what the individual saw or what they heard, smelled and even may have tasted, but it's their perception of what happened to them or what they saw and what they heard. There is a picture forever painted in the recesses of their mind of what happened that represents to them a point of no return. The images are so solidified within the memory of the happening that the mind has to take action to try to process an understanding of what just occurred, but it can't. The vivid colors of red blood, bodies that are blue because the breath is no longer within the dead corpse, and the sight of broken bones as often seen in war or an accident are imprinted on the mind's eye.

Remember the story about three blind men trying to describe an elephant? The first blind man is feeling the animal's tusk and he thinks it is long, smooth, hard like a bone, and tapers at the end. The second blind man feels the side of the giant mammal and thinks it is huge like a wall blocking one's way. The third blind man feels the tail and his perception is it is long like a rope. Even this story has a different variation depending on the culture telling it. An experience that we have seen or experienced is processed through our perception of the event in many different ways. Ten people may have seen the same horror and you will have ten different views on what was seen and what occurred.

There's a song that says, "What doesn't kill you makes you stronger." Obviously that song is very wrong. People survive many situations of horror, but they do not come out on the other side stronger. Oftentimes, they come out on the other side physically broken, emotionally shattered, mentally defeated, and spiritually fragmented. They may be so physically damaged that they are not able to move or breathe without the assistance of a caregiver and machines to breathe for them. How does that make you stronger? How is one made stronger when what they have witnessed or experienced is so devastating that their mind can't comprehend what happened to them and it shuts down? That person becomes catatonic. How is one's strength made stronger when they are lost and stumbling around in a spiritual void and they can't see the light of salvation? NO, what doesn't kill does not make you stronger!

PSALM 23:4, ESV

Even though I walk through the valley of the shadow of death, I will fear no evil, for you are with me; your rod and your staff, they comfort me.

You may, indeed, feel as though you are walking through the valley of death while you are experiencing an especially strong phobic episode. How do we replace fear with faith? What is faith?

According to the Nuttall encyclopedia: *Faith in its proper spiritual sense and meaning is a deep-rooted belief affecting the whole life, that the visible universe in every section of it, particularly here and now, rests on and is the manifestation of an eternal and an unchangeable Unseen Power, whose name is Good, or God.*

A big factor of having faith means recognizing that you have no control over anything at all. You realize that there is a greater power, whether it be God, the universe, or a belief in good vs. evil. Faith means letting go of your worries, your fears, feeling peace in knowing that your life has purpose and that you will be fine in the end. To have faith means to recognize that the world does not revolve around you. You know that there are so many variables that factor into a human life that you could never have control over any part of it and letting go of imagined control will be okay.

We are told in Hebrews 11:1: Now faith is confidence in what we hope for and assurance about what we do not see.

The definition of hope is a feeling of optimism or a desire that something will happen. Once we are able to feel hopeful, we will feel like we are coming out of the cold darkness of fear into the embracing warmth of reassurance. Hope is the opposite side of the coin of fear. Maintaining hopefulness takes effort on our part, but the results of maintaining hope are worth the effort. Faith will keep us in a frame of mind that allows our dreams to become a reality, to give us a future and a vision of desires obtained.

The Angel of Hope gives one the strength to keep going in the face of distress and prevents us from falling into the valley of the shadow of death. The Angel of Hope perseveres with us and fuels our determination to survive. The Angel of Hope at times is our lifeline and salvation when all else fails.

The Angel of Hope fuels us with divine love. Hope creates a new space for the gift of hope and for success, hope for a better world for ourselves and loved ones, hope for a peace of mind, and hope for less strife. When we add action to our hope, we change the hopeless situation into a new beginning for everyone.

The Angel of Hope assists us in using the power of hope in new positive ways: we become a source of nourishment when we are in a trial of life and to become a cocreator in the manifestation of a more harmonious world.

PRAYER

I call upon my guardian angel and the Angel of Hope to walk with me through the valley of fear. Help me to observe the situation at hand and to see it through new eyes by inspiring me to take loving action in correcting my view of the event at hand.

Help me to feel the vibration of hope lifting me higher to have the strength to face any obstacles that might be in my path of life. I ask that the Angel of Hope show me the faith I need to see that the universe is working out the highest good for me and everyone involved in every situation. I ask the Angel of Hope to instill in me the knowledge that my needs will be met in all situations.

I give thanks for this power to see the good in every situation. I give thanks for the lessons I needed to learn during this time of stress. I give thanks to the Angel of Hope for the inspiration to see the plan for higher consciousness of peace and harmony that is accepted by love.

Guilt, bitterness, fear; they can be devastating emotions that can cripple us. These emotions also have a counterpart that is just as devastating: rejection.

Children often feel rejected by one or both parents. Sometimes the feelings of rejection are imagined, but other times they are very real and demonstrated in the family setting. The pain these children feel as they grow into adults can leave an emotional scar that some may never heal from. If feelings of exclusion are not dealt with, the adult-child may become a bitter and angry individual.

4

It Hurts When a Parent Rejects a Child

"It hurts to know my mother did not want me," Elizabeth began. "She always liked my brother better than me." Elizabeth grew up feeling rejected by her mother. Many of us have felt the sting of rejection. As a typical-looking middle-aged woman, Elizabeth feels invisible and as though she does not count. Elizabeth's self-esteem has been stunted through the years. She has found herself stuck in moving forward and in realizing her own self-worth. Elizabeth has experienced pain throughout her life because she and her mother never bonded.

"I felt I was not good enough and no matter how hard I tried it did not matter. I never seemed to measure up," Elizabeth said, blinking back tears.

"My brother had the best clothes, the best grades, the best of everything. He did not do anything to help around the house. What he wanted came first. I felt like I was standing outside looking in through the window at the people inside of the house. I never really felt like I belonged. I did not feel like I was part of my own family. I felt like I was an intruder in the wrong house."

When one sibling is placed in the spotlight, the others suffer. The siblings who can't measure up often have feelings of frustration and despair. He or she feels hopeless. As a result depression may become a problem even as a child. Their world is gray and bleak, void of any colors of passionate pink or joyful yellow that come with the love of a parent for their child.

At times, a rebuffed sibling may become overbearing and their discouragement may show up by misbehaving. They will act out at times to get their parents' attention. Any attention is better than none at all. Or some children will withdraw into themselves becoming invisible. These children have no identity of who they are and no feelings of self-worth and importance. It is almost like they never existed at all. They walk through life and are invisible to everyone, including themselves.

"I decided when I had children I would show them how much I love them," Elizabeth said. "I was not about to play favorites."

Family relationships are often strained between the parents and the shunned child. Misunderstandings are many and often go unresolved. If the misunderstandings are not recognized and dealt with, the same problems can arise in the next generation.

"I love my boys so very much, but there is a strain between my youngest son and me," Elizabeth said. "He complains I can't accept him as he is. He says he feels like an outsider in his own family."

Elizabeth's son has voiced the feelings she had as a child. These emotions still plague Elizabeth as an adult. Elizabeth seems to be living through her childhood frustrations once again, only this time with her son.

"I was rejected by my mother and now my own son is rejecting me. I do not understand it. I have never played favorites with my boys. But once again, no matter what I do it is not good enough."

"My son says I am overbearing and I should stay out of his life. He says I should mind my own business."

"I do not feel like I try to run his life. When I see he is going to make a mistake, I try to point it out, but he gets angry. I feel like I am living in a vicious cycle."

What happened to Elizabeth? Why is Elizabeth having the same problem with her son that she had with her mother? Why is she experiencing the same emotions she had as a child?

Elizabeth felt abandoned by her mother. Feeling abandoned made Elizabeth feel undesired, left behind, insecure, and discarded. At times, Elizabeth thought that it would have been better had she never been born. Elizabeth was determined not to make the same mistake with her children as her mother had made with her. But Elizabeth's perception of herself has caused low self-esteem and has carried over into her adulthood, causing her to project her feelings onto her son.

"I did not make the same mistake with my son of showing favoritism, but I made the mistake of being overbearing. As a result, my son felt he could not do anything right. He was frustrated and felt rejected. He turned away from me. When this happened, I had the same feelings of rejection I had as a child. I still struggle with rejection as an adult."

Elizabeth's husband is a very kind man with a great deal of patience and insight. Don tried to help Elizabeth see how her actions with their son was affecting not only her relationship with their son, but also with the family as a whole.

"It took Don a long time to get through to me. The day he said, 'Elizabeth, you have got to stop being so overbearing. You are overidentifying with our son. It hurts me to see your relationship with our son so strained.' Don's words hit me hard, but they finally began to penetrate into my heart and mind," Elizabeth confessed.

Elizabeth began to open up her heart and listened to what Don had to say.

"It was painful to hear how people saw me. I wanted to help, but in reality I was sticking my nose in other people's business. I was making my son feel stonewalled by trying to get him to conform to my way of thinking."

Don helped Elizabeth see that by telling their son what to do in every situation, she was making him feel he was not competent enough to make his own decisions. She was eroding his self-esteem by her interference in his life.

"My interfering in my son's life made him feel like I thought he was not capable of making his own choices. He had the same feelings I had as a child. He did not feel he could please me and his self-esteem was low. The cycle was continuing. I decided the cycle had to be broken."

How did Elizabeth break the cycle?

"I had to realize my son is an individual and not an extension of myself," Elizabeth started.

By seeing her son as an individual, Elizabeth began to see her son as the person he truly is. Also, by seeing her son as a person in his own right, Elizabeth began to understand that her son's decisions were his responsibility, not hers.

"I do not always like his choices, but I am realizing he has his own path to walk. What I want for him may not be God's plan for him."

When Elizabeth's son decided to move to another state, she felt deserted and abandoned once again.

"I like having my family close by."

Don helped Elizabeth to see that their son was not deserting her, but following his own path.

"My son seemed to move farther away from me. I felt like I was losing him. But Don helped me to see I was wanting my way and what was best for me, not what was best for our son. I was smothering him instead of mothering him."

Elizabeth soon learned by letting go of her son and letting him become the man he is intended to be, instead of trying to control him, she soon discovered that her relationship with her son was improving. They began to talk and not be at odds.

"I learned a child can feel lonely when a parent is overbearing. I know a child can feel neglected when a parent shows favoritism. In both cases the child is made to feel he is not accepted as an individual. The child is made to feel incompetent and worthless."

It was a very long and hard struggle for Elizabeth to let go of control issues she had developed through the years. Elizabeth discovered that her overidentification was also a form of playing favorites on an unconscious level. By learning this she was able to start working through her feelings of being estranged from her son. It is human nature to want to be in control of our life. We live with the false assumption that we are in control, however, this is just a false illusion. We simply cannot be in control of everything or everyone around us, this is the lesson that we have to learn. The physical world cannot be controlled, so the task before us is to learn to manage what is inside of us, our thoughts and responses to the external world. Our thoughts and emotions are a reflection of how we deal with the outside world.

Struggle seems to be a never-ending pattern of disappointment we bring on ourselves as we attempt to control our lives through external means. We drive ourselves crazy by trying to manipulate events in our lives to make the perfect decision on every single event. It does not really matter which choice we make, the important thing to realize is why we made the decision we did. That is where the real power to influence our life comes from, in our reasoning in how we came to make the decision that was made.

Once we learn about what motivates us to make certain choices, we began to learn about the character of our spirit. We learn that our choices are made either through fear or through faith. The outcome of each decision is determined on the source of energy we use in determining the course of action we will take. Are we using fear-based negative energy? In doing so, we are giving away our power to try to create a positive outcome. If our decision is based on faith, then we are using our power to create a positive outcome in our life. The reflection of every decision is to some extent based in either fear or faith.

"I did not know what a wonderful person my son was until I began to look at him as an individual. Sometimes it has to hurt before we can grow. But the most important thing is, is that we do grow. If we do not grow, we die on the inside and wither up as a vine would in a drought," Elizabeth said as she shared her new-found wisdom.

The root cause of rejection is actually rather simple. Damaged self-esteem comes from the result of a misplaced identity. Rejection can elicit emotional pain so sharp that it affects our thinking, it overwhelms us with the blood red anger that erodes our confidence and self-esteem. It destabilizes our fundamental feeling of belonging. We are no longer grounded in family and community.

Whenever we base our identity on someone else's thoughts about who we are, we make ourselves vulnerable to the damage of rejection. Many of us will base our identity on what our parents, teachers, or friends think of us. We have set ourselves up for failure when we look to others to define our self-worth. It is our responsibility to define who we are. We are not to place restrictions on defining our self-worth by saying, "I am worthy as long as I have the love of my parent, my partner . . ."

With rejection comes a mixture of trust and mistrust in a child's basic social attitudes that is crucial in developing a healthy personality. A belief in the trustworthiness of others sets the stage for positive interactions. Doubts about trusting normally arise under circumstances such as broken promises. For most individuals broken promises or betrayed trust is usually temporary and circumscribed. However, if the inability to establish a trusting relationship arises, then there is a potential problem. Under these situations a person may lose self-esteem and feel vey unsure of themselves and may have a pronounced distortion in one's ability to relate to others.

Trust is necessary to interact successfully with others. One has to trust their self-interpretation of the words spoken and the meaning behind them during interactions with others.

We need to remember that we are created in the image of God. If we are created in His image, then why are we looking to mankind to define our self-value? Our God has defined our value when He brought us into His house and made us His children. His love alone makes us valued and worthwhile. He-Who-Is-Good does not reject us and He does not diminish our self-esteem by rejecting us. We are His and we will always be His.

Do you know rejection attaches itself on physical pain pathways in the brain? MRI studies show that the same areas of the brain become activated when we experience rejection just as when we experience physical pain. This is the scientific proof why rejection hurts so much.

Yes, it hurts and the devastating pain runs deep within our soul. But it feels so good when we do grow from the hurt. Unless we face the legitimate pain in our lives, we will not grow. If we do not grow from the physical suffering or discomfort caused by our reaction to rejection, we risk becoming and staying neurotically conflicted. When this happens, we become severely handicapped both emotionally and spiritually.

Strategies to overcome rejection:

1. Acknowledge your emotions. Do not try to ignore or suppress how you feel. It doesn't work and it will only fester until you do acknowledge your feelings.
2. Treat yourself with compassion. If you can't be compassionate with yourself, how can you possibly show real compassion to others?
3. Refuse to let rejection define who you are. Do not take on the belief that you are not worthwhile because of another

person's actions. Their beliefs are erroneous and have no bearing on your self-worth. In reality, their thoughts are just that, theirs alone and really none of your business.

4. Learn from the experience. Learn to define who you are based on the facts that you are a worthwhile individual. You are your own person and your thoughts about yourself are the only thoughts that matter, so beware of your thoughts.

Elizabeth learned some strategies in overcoming her sense of rejection and low self-esteem. She read self-help books and articles, learning how to move out of her feelings of being dejected. She became involved in activities that gave her a sense of accomplishment. Elizabeth likes to read and learned about a reading program at the local schools for volunteers to read to the children. Elizabeth volunteered to read books to the children at the local schools and for the library's children's storytime program. In doing this, Elizabeth discovered the joy in helping a child who was having difficulties with reading. She helped the children to realize that they too could read. Seeing the delight in the eyes of the children as she read to them helped Elizabeth realize that she was making a child's day a little happier. Hearing the children calling out her name in excited anticipation as she walked into the classroom made Elizabeth feel excited as well.

Elizabeth learned that if she stepped out of her comfort zone and looked at activities she had not tried before, she was opening herself up to new opportunities. Elizabeth volunteered to write letters for residents in one of the local nursing homes. Elizabeth felt a closeness to the residents and learned that her interaction with them formed new friendships. These friendships she would hold very dear to her, cherishing the time she had with her new found friends. To Elizabeth's surprise, her self-esteem began to grow stronger.

Most importantly, Elizabeth learned that the only approval she needs is her own self-approval. She learned not to see herself from other peoples' eyes, but from her own self-perspective. No one knows her as well as she knows her own self and she learned that her perspective is the only one that matters. Other people do not know the full story of her heart and they are looking through clouded glasses of distortion.

Elizabeth soon began to make short-term goals, then midterm goals, and long-term goals on things that she wanted to achieve. She learned in setting goals and reaching those goals that her self-esteem grew as she accomplishment these objectives. She started with smaller intentions such as reading to the children for story time and realized her own self-worth as she gave back to her community.

Elizabeth also learned to look beyond herself and focus on what was going on in the world around her. In doing this, Elizabeth was able to get out of her own way and move forward in life. Once she learned to stop dwelling on the past rejections she felt as a child, she began to feel the light and warmth, the sunny yellow that joy and the peace that life has to offer if we will just look beyond ourselves. She learned to embrace the wonderful person she is.

Elizabeth now knows the pleasures of unselfish joy and happiness that one finds in service to others. She also knows the self-satisfying pleasure and peace of mind that come with self-respect.

Emotional abandonment is a subjective emotional state in which people feel undesired, left behind, insecure, or discarded. People experiencing emotional desertion may feel at a loss or feel like they have been thrown away without a second thought being given to their very existence. They feel cut off from a life source of support that has been withdrawn. They feel abandoned and left behind. This support was either suddenly removed, or withdrawn through a process of slow detection. To be left behind leaves one feeling rejected, which is a significant component of emotional abandonment. It causes a biological impact in that it activates the physical pain centers in the brain. When this happens it can leave an emotional scar on the brain's warning system.

When a child feels deserted, they are emotionally starved, they long to be loved and need to have the emptiness on the inside filled up with belonging to a family. Emotional emptiness is a tragedy and leads to suicidal tendencies. This emptiness invokes a sense of profound hopelessness, extreme loneliness, and a feeling of being unloved, abused, and neglected. According to the *New York Times*, teen suicide increased from 6.3 percent in 2009 to 7.8 percent in 2011. These children are emotionally disturbed and starved of affection and love. These children have no one to turn to for guidance, love, and support. They have no one to embrace them in love and to make them feel like they are worthwhile. This is a tragedy that our civilization must address.

Emotional needs of a child include:

~ to be listened to and understood,
~ to be nurtured,
~ to be appreciated,
~ to be valued,
~ to be accepted,
~ to know affection,
~ to be loved, and
~ to have companionship and support so they can develop trust,

Trust is related to faith in the goodness of the human nature. This approach assumes that people are basically kind and considerate in most situations.

If a person has experienced broken promises and trust throughout their childhood, they may begin to mistrust people in general. This mental state is laced with the basic assumptions that are brimming with suspicions about being able to understand and predict possible outcomes. Interactions are difficult when the outcomes of interpersonal relationships have been validated time and time again.

The foundations of trust are tested throughout a child's development. These foundations can be reestablished and renewed with each new crisis and conflict that has positive results. As a child experiences positive outcomes, they are able to express their own feelings freely, in an honest and forthcoming manner. Emotions can be shown in an acceptable manner that strengthens how the child feels in a given situation.

A healthy and trusting person recognizes spiritually that acceptance is a natural part of their experience that provides meaning to life. For the person who knows trust, it can be reaffirmation of a sense of belonging to a higher power. During stressful times an emotionally healthy person will seek their spiritual connection for support and guidance.

Our most precious treasures of life are our relationships with other people, especially those with whom we love. Our relationships inspire us to be better people and nourish our spirit. As humans, we need the companionship so our soul will thrive in love and affection.

Sometimes a relationship will deteriorate because of a misunderstanding or complex circumstances. At times, we see what we want to see in a situation rather than what is really there.

What it boils down to is how we truly see ourselves. Do we have self-respect? Do we love ourselves? How we see ourselves determines the quality of life that we will have. The truth is, if we do not have a healthy relationship with ourselves, we will not be capable of making healthy decisions concerning any aspect of our life. If we are making choices out of fear, we are giving away our power to control our own destiny to others to make the decision for us. Is that what you really want, to have others make the decision on what direction your life will take? I certainly hope not! You have to take hold of the reins of your life and guide it as you see fit.

When we choose to live in spirit instead of the illusions of the physical world, we map out the direction we will take in life. Every time we choose to acknowledge the power of spirit over the illusion of this 3D world, we have given power to our inner soul's energy field and when this happens we gain strength and enhance our internal power. As we fortify our energy field, we are better equipped to block out negative people who will try to drain our energy. We have to protect ourselves from energy vampires. You know who those people are, they are the ones who keep you in a despairing and exhausting state of feeling drained. They are the ones who just suck the life right out of you.

Intuition is defined as the ability to understand something immediately, without the need for conscious reasoning. Once we connect with our intuitive instincts we are better able to make decisions by being grounded into the here and now. By being in the present moment, we are able to use the information we have to access our intuitive reasoning and make better decisions and have positive results.

Developing self-esteem requires that we have to work to discover who we are. We have to learn which emotions are driving us before we can learn to do the driving. It is not easy to take a look at our secrets that we hide from others and more importantly the ones we strive to hide from ourselves. It takes courage to look at our shadow side, to examine the darkness within ourselves. It takes more courage to acknowledge who we are and the positive contributions we have to offer to the world. Why is it so hard to love ourselves? When and where do we draw the line on self-criticism?

Developing self-esteem requires one to become radical and to cause a revolution to turn your world upside-down and inside-out, to create your identity both within your soul and outside of yourself in the physical world. It will be hard to separate from our group's core beliefs on who they think we are or who they think we should be. It will be extremely difficult to cut the cords that keep us tied to our family's belief of who they think we are, but it has to be done if we want to move forward to free ourselves from the group energy that has kept us tied to them and bogged down. Our group will resist in letting us sever the energetic cord. It has to be done and must be done for us to break free and become the spiritual beings we are intended to be. We have to create our own voice and speak our own truth.

As we develop this inner strength, find our own voice, and speak our own truth, we are able to reach Spiritual Maturity. As we develop our Spiritual Maturity, we begin to replace the influences of our group and others who want to influence and control us. We have to ask ourselves, "What do I believe? What do I think?"

As we assess our external world and begin to better know who we are, we then turn inward to assess our relationship with our Creator God. This self-examination of our relationship with God gives us strength to handle the consequences of self-exploration of our thoughts. During this phase of self-discovery, we may find that we need to withdraw for a period of rest, recovery, and healing.

The next step in Spiritual Maturity is one of becoming self-centered. Since self-exploration and development is taking place, we are in a sense creating a new image of who we are. To be self-centered has two meanings. The first is the most common definition of putting one's self first and the second is that of becoming centered within yourself and grounded into the energy of Creator Source. It is in the second definition of self-centered we are focused on. Yes, there are times that we have to put ourselves first in order to survive. We have to learn to set boundaries with others who are not happy with the changes we are going through and who are not happy with our spiritual maturity.

The last stage of our development in self-esteem is internal. It is one of determining what your principles are, standing in your dignity and faith without compromising who you have become and who you intend to be. As your own spirit and strength takes hold, the rest of the world and your family and friends will yield to its force and energy. Honor yourself and others will honor you. Respect yourself and you will soon see others respecting you as well. Embrace who you now are and continue on your journey to Spiritual Maturity.

The Angel of Relationships can raise our perspective to see circumstances from a different point of view. The Angel of Relationships can ensure a greater understanding and appreciation of others.

PRAYER

I ask the Angel of Relationships and my guardian angel to surround me so that I can see the happy images of people I know and to see the truth as it arises within me. Let me see the truth that these people love and care deeply about me. Let them see that I have a profound love for them.

I am open to a new understanding of my relationships and my role in them. The Angel of Relationships shows me a vast network of people who care about me with the most loving respect. I contemplate on how they have touched my life. I am filled with the deepest gratitude for all of these individuals. I ask the Angel of Relationships to guide me to higher levels of understanding. I ask that the Angel of Relationships shows me the highest good for the individuals in my life and for myself.

I give praise to Father God for the blessings of these loved ones in my life. I pray that I will be a blessing to them as I open my heart to those around me.

When we experience pain, we often wonder: Does God understand? How can he understand? After all, He is God, and God has never had the problems we have. Or has He?

5

How Do I Find Trust Again?

" I just do not think God understands," Stan said as he shook his head. "Stars were out in full force. The moon was bright and full that night. You could smell spring in the air. Everything was blooming and you could feel the renewed life after the long months of cold winter gales. But my life had just been shattered. June, my wife, told me she was leaving."

Stan is a third-generation farmer. Stan is a tall, rugged, and sturdy man. He takes pride in his farm. Being an outdoor person, Stan enjoys the smell of freshly plowed soil. He enjoys being close to nature and hard work does not bother him.

"I have never been ashamed of being a farmer. It makes me feel good to look out over a good crop and know my grain is feeding people from all walks of life. I knew I wanted to be a farmer and I was glad to finish college. I was eager to put my newly learned knowledge to work."

But Stan's wife, June, did not look at farming as a source of pride. The lack of prestige and isolation were more than she could bear.

"I put my trust in my wife and her refusal of my love hurt me. June let lust for the fast life enter her heart. Soon, she was having several affairs. This went on for eight years. I tried to help her see the goodness of the country life. I even looked the other way and was willing to forgive her for the affairs," Stan said, sadly.

June turned her back on Stan and moved out.

"I liked being married and when June moved out, I became fearful. I realized I would be facing life alone and the thought scared me. I do not mind being alone, but being left to go through life alone is another story," Stan said.

Stan liked sharing his life with June. He wanted someone there to share his hopes and dreams. The thought of living by himself and not having the support of a wife depressed Stan. The thought of not having children to see come into this world and love was also a loss for Stan. He had wanted to have children and see them growing up on the farm. He wanted to have heirs to leave the farm to and to keep the farm in the family. He wanted to see the next generation taking care of the land.

Stan began to feel God did not understand how badly he was hurting. How could He understand? His life is perfect.

"One day while I was working and feeling sorry for myself, God the Father, touched my heart," Stan recalls. "I was thinking about how hurt I was from June's deceptions and desertion. God could not understand this kind of pain. How could He, He is the Almighty? How could God know the pain of rejection? Slowly, it came to me that our Creator did understand rejection. June lusted for the fast life, turning her back on my way of life. Man lusted for the things of the world and walked away from Jesus."

The realization that God did understand how Stan felt began to turn Stan around. The moment when Stan suddenly had a profound awareness that God was speaking to him was his moment of truth. In that moment, Stan wanted to know everything about God. Stan suddenly found himself wanting to know His Savior on a deeper level, there was a thirst that could not be quenched, this was the turning point for Stan.

Stan realized that as he was going through this difficult time, his knowing God would help him react to these trying times with a different perspective and with a strength that is not his own. Stan saw that no problem has the capacity to be insurmountable to Father God. Source is greater than all the problems that will come into our life, and Father will not leave us alone to deal with them.

When we are suffering, God is involved in our suffering with us. God has created humanity with the ability to choose. He has given us freewill. This means that we are not forced into a relationship with Him. Creator allows us to reject Him and to commit to other paths in life as well. He cannot force us to be loving. He cannot force us to be good. That would be a violation of our freewill. God knows the pain and suffering we encounter in this world. He experienced it through Jesus as Jesus hung on the cross.

"Once when I was thinking about being alone, I realized that our ever-loving Father understood that fear also. Creator is alone in the sense that He is the only perfect being. He understands man's aloneness. That is why He created woman. He also felt fear with Jesus, as Christ faced the cross alone."

But the Son was not alone and neither was Stan. I AM THAT I AM helped Stan by showing him that He would always be by Stan's side and help him through tough times. Gradually, Stan's heart felt the healing warmth and love in knowing God did understand.

"Knowing that Universal Love is there to help me through the difficult times in life gives me the strength to hold on. Our Father will never let me face any situation alone. He will always be there to help me cope with life's blows. All I have to do is ask."

Three years after June moved out, Stan's father suddenly died.

"As I buried my dad, I knew God would help me. Dad's death was sudden and unexpected. His death was a blow to the family. His death illuminated the frightening reality of how fragile we really are," Stan says.

"God knows the pain that death brings. He saw the body of Jesus hanging on the cross as the shadow of death approached. He saw the terrible suffering Jesus went through."

Christ once said, "I am the Way, and the Truth and the Life" (John 14:6 NIV). This promise to show us the way and to be with us is enough to help us through the hard times.

"My grandmother once told me, 'Life is much like a rose. Velvet softness of the delicate petals let us know just how precious life is. Rich deep colors show us how rich life can be with God as our caretaker. The beauty of life can fill one with wonders, but the thorns of reality are there to remind us that without God, there is no beauty, no life.' She was right," Stan said with a new understanding.

How does one deal with being rejected in love? How do you work through this type of abandonment? We are most vulnerable when we are in love and even more so when we are rejected in love. Being rejected in love is devastating and we feel we will not recover and we feel like we have been "thrown away".

One of the hardest areas to be shunned is in romantic love. The suffering that comes with this type of unreceptive love is considerably harder than in most other types of love. Interestingly, many people tend to love and desire those who are not as passionate about them. It seems like being discarded or merely the fear of being thrown out makes us more passionate about what we can't have, making us suffer even more. You may find yourself feeling lonely and isolated, lost.

Researchers have found that physical pain and intense emotional pain, such as feelings of rejection after a romantic breakup activate the same pain receptors that process pathways in the brain. Researchers also say that the results suggest that pain and social rejection may have overlapping sensory mechanisms in the brain. If this is true, this is the reason that we actually feel pain after a romantic breakup. Research shows that the brain's mu-opioid receptor system releases natural painkillers, or opioids, in response to social pain. This is the same neurological system that releases opioids during times of physical pain.

When you first realize you are being rejected, you may be unable to speak and you feel physically ill. Physical symptoms and other symptoms such as being unable to sleep, work, or concentrate can persist for several weeks. The intensity of negative emotions will gradually fade, although you will definitely continue having good days and bad days for a while. (6)

You have to remember, our emotions and how we react to them are a decision that we consciously make. We are not left helpless to our emotions, we do have control over how we will manage our response in situations. I know that at the time of extreme stress this may not seem to be the truth. It seems as though we are left helpless in the situation. It feels like we have no control over our emotional reaction during the events being played out.

Here are some practical tips on how to deal with rejection, ease pain, and make your recovery period significantly shorter:

~ Tell yourself it will go away, because it will. Keep reminding yourself that this is only temporary. You may be even thankful for this experience in the future. Remember, "This too shall pass."

~ Engage in physical activities. Physical activity forces us to concentrate outside of ourselves and live in the moment. This is the reason why we feel so alive when we are active, and this is the reason why exercise can be actually addictive.

~ Focus outside of yourself. Although it might be hard to do during the first stage of being excluded, avoid blaming and criticizing yourself. Be your own best friend. If you catch yourself analyzing your past or yourself, acknowledge the feeling, then gradually draw attention away from yourself to something external.

~ Learn something new. Learning a new skill can be challenging; it helps us to heal by keeping us busy and focused. To make things even better, learning a new skill may help you discover new opportunities or meet new people.

~ Travel. New places are always fun to explore, and just like the suggestions above, new places will distract our attention from negative thoughts and add excitement to your life.

~ Meet new people. When you meet someone new, you want to put your best foot forward, and this will force you to pick yourself up. New people have new exciting stories to tell which helps you stay distracted.

~ Use self-hypnosis. Hypnosis helps you access the unconscious mind and shape it in ways you never dreamed were possible.

~ Consider counseling or online counseling. We all know professional counseling works, but having to book an appointment and then actually go to the clinic may seem overwhelming. You might be not in a good shape, and you might fear that, by going there, you'll embarrass yourself in front of strangers. Online counseling offers all benefits of traditional counseling without the anxiety associated with going to see your therapist.(6)

Consider consulting a life coach. A life coach can provide you with the drive and guidance to help you improve your career, your relationships, and your life. A life coach can help you recognize your skills, your dreams, to help you refocus your life's goals, and to move past the challenges that stand in your way of reaching these goals.

John 1:11 ESV: "He came to his own, and his own people did not receive him."

Jesus was rejected by his own family, by his own people. Jesus said to them, "Only in his hometown, among his relatives and in his own house is a prophet without honor." Mark 6:4 NIV

Jesus knew the sting of rejection. He felt the pain just as we do. Jesus, however, was able to turn to God for strength. So are we able to turn to God for strength.

God tells us in Jeremiah 29:11 that He has plans for us to prosper and give us hope and a future.

Rejection works so subtly and covertly to destroy your self-esteem and causes you to feel sorry for yourself. Nonacceptance spurs you to reject other people before they have an opportunity to abandon you. You isolate yourself from those around you who want to show you love and support.

To move beyond the pain of exclusion, pray for the individual who caused you emotional pain. Make a conscious decision to move forward and release the despair felt with being brushed off, and dismissed by the one you loved.

While making the attempt to move forward, imagine within your mind's eye meeting with the person who rejected your love. Meet with this person in a neutral place in your imagination. Invite them in to talk with you. Extend your hand in friendship. By offering your hand in friendship, you are making an impression on your subconscious mind that you are ready to move forward and let go of the circumstances that lead to your heartache. Tell this person how you felt when you met them and how you felt when they spurned your love. Tell them of your desire to end the relationship as friends instead of having hard feelings. By taking this step, you are forgiving this person for hurting you and wishing them well on their journey in life. By showing this person compassion and grace, you are being compassionate and graceful with yourself.

Refuse to belittle yourself over someone else's shortsightedness. Sometimes, a relationship just is not meant to be. You may have had more of a heartache by being in the relationship; oil and water just do not mix.

Accept your uniqueness. This is a good opportunity to eliminate toxic people from your life. We cannot be a friend to everyone we meet and Source does not expect us to try to befriend certain people.

Make sure that you have recovered from the last relationship before you start a new one. You can't truly have a successful relationship with another person until you reconcile with what happened in the last one. When we jump from one relationship into another one without analyzing what went wrong in the last one, we are setting ourselves up for another heartbreak.

If we do not deal with the problems in our current involvement, we will make the same mistakes in future romantic situations. Until we learn from the previous mistakes, we will be grounded in the same frustration and we will not be able to move forward in life. We have to learn the lessons in each unique meeting or we will keep running into the same encounters until we do learn the lesson that we were intended to learn.

I do not know about you, but I do not relish the thought of having to repeat the same encounters until I learn the lesson that was presented to me in the first place. Being held in a continuously repeating loop to learn a lesson seems a bit harsh to me. I would rather learn it the first time around and move on.

Listen to your intuition when entering into a new relationship. Do not try to make something happen. If this is the person you are intended to be with, then the events will unfold as they should. See the truth in all situations. Do not overlook any red flags that might appear as you get to know this new person.

When the needs for a relationship are met, you will find that you are more creative, rational, and logical. You are better able to solve problems.

Feeling alone can be painful. Having a relationship with your Higher Power offers support and will give you confidence to explore new friendships. Building a social network is important in moving forward in life. This network can give you the support and feedback in social situations that will help build your confidence. Prayer and meditation establish a bridge to alleviate feelings of alienation.

Eventually, Stan was able to move forward in his life. He learned that he had to love himself before he could truly love another. Stan had looked to June to prove his self-worth instead of looking to Source to show him that he is loved. Stan learned that to love oneself is not selfishness, but necessary to be emotionally healthy. Stan learned that unconditional love starts with ALL-THAT-THERE-IS and once we accept His love, then we are able to extend this love to others.

Most of our prayers are pleas for healing. When we call on the Angel of Healing for help, we are assisted in the goal to heal every area of our life. The request for healing can be for physical healing, emotional restoration, or healing of the spirit. The need to be healed supersedes all other desires.

True healing first comes from the soul. Our soul is connected to our physical, emotional, and mental bodies. It is our desire to be whole and aligned in all areas of life. It is our desire to be complete.

All thoughts are a prayer that projects energy out into the universe and sets into motion what we are thinking about. When we strive to lift our thoughts to merge with the mind of God, and focus our thoughts on healing with grace, we will then become the light of the Divine. This light will radiate back to us bringing a healing and wholeness. When we are joined with the divine light, the highest good will always manifest for us the perfect solution for our needs.

PRAYER

I ask that the Angel of Healing and my guardian angel assist me in seeing the Truth in this situation that is in need of healing energy. I ask that the Angel of Healing take me to the healing room to be attended to by my angels of health.

I see the light of the Great Healer and Archangel Raphael surrounding me and enveloping me in their energies of health. As I am filled with this light of perfect health, it radiates from within me outward for the rest of the world to see and to receive. I fix my eyes on the Creator of life and give thanks of humble gratitude to the healing that has been given to me for my highest good.

God does understand us. He understands us and stands by us. But there are times when we feel God's absence. Why is this? Is it because of something we did? Maybe it's something we didn't do.

During times like this we may feel hurt and confused. We may even feel angry at God for not letting us feel his presence. After all, didn't he say he would be there to help us through difficult times? If this is true, why is it that we ask, "Where are you God?"

6

The Illusion:
Isolation from God

"Where are you God? Where were you when my son was hurt? Why do I only feel your absence? Why don't you answer me?" Sara demanded.

"Seeing my son lying on the surgical cart brought a pain that stabbed me to the very core of my soul," Sara began. "It took all my strength to hold back the tears and try to comfort Joseph before they took him back to surgery. He was only seven years old and so afraid."

Three weeks before, Joseph had fallen at school. As a result, he developed a large hematoma that would not dissolve. To complicate matters, Joseph has hemophilia.

"My son's hemophilia is a mild form and he has not had to be infused with the cryoprecipitate on a regular basis. Joseph only had the product once in his life, at eighteen months old before a scheduled surgery. Cryoprecipitate is the agent given to some hemophiliacs to aid in the clotting of their blood. I thanked the Almighty often that we did not have to worry about getting AIDS from the clotting agent. Cryoprecipitate is made from blood. Many hemophiliacs have gotten AIDS from the very treatment they needed to save their lives. I guess I even became a little overconfident in my relationship with God," Sara confessed.

AIDS stands for "acquired immunodeficiency syndrome." AIDS is an advanced stage of the infection with the human immunodeficiency virus (HIV). People with AIDS have weakened immune systems that make them vulnerable to selected conditions and infections. Human immunodeficiency virus infection is a disease in which there is a severe loss of the body's cellular immunity, greatly lowering the resistance to infection and malignancy. AIDS can be transmitted through sexual contact with an infected person, by transmission through pregnancy from an infected mother to her unborn child, coming in contact with contaminated blood, and needle sticks from carriers of AIDS. Many hemophiliac children acquired AIDS from the blood products that they need to clot their blood before the testing on the blood products could detect the AIDS virus.

Sara had been a nurse for thirteen years, but it did not help ease Sara's fears. If anything, her knowledge about medical procedures and her experience as a nurse in the medical field only increased her fears. Sara had comforted many families when their children were going to have a surgical procedure. But, on this day no one was there to give support to Sara.

"I was a pediatric nurse for ten years and I had reassured a lot of parents who had children going back to surgery and tried to calm their fears, but no one was there to reassure me. Not even my Father's presence was felt. I was afraid and alone during my son's surgery."

Fear became more pronounced after surgery as Joseph had to be given cryoprecipitate before and after surgery.

"Blood was drawn a few weeks after surgery to test for the HIV and AIDS virus. The time waiting on getting the test results back was a nightmare. I had to wait several days for the results. I feared my son's death. I trusted Creator God, yet I felt He had turned his back on me," recalled Sara.

Sara's fear turned into rage. She resented the situation.

"I was so angry with people who were spreading the AIDS virus. This resentment was such a new experience for me, and I did not know how to work through it. I became angry with God, too. I fussed and yelled at Him every day."

Father God had always been with Sara. She did not have a big conversion or a dramatic conversion. He had just always been with her. Even as a child she knew God's presence and had always talked with Him.

But with her son's injury, Sara did not have the comfort she had always known. She felt as if Source had turned His back on her.

"I yelled at Creator God and demanded to know where He was. I wanted to know why He was doing this. I felt as if He had forsaken me. This made me angry because I felt I did not deserve to be left alone during this time of crisis," Sara said.

Confusion in the turnaround in her relationship with Creator caused Sara to search for an answer. Reading about Job helped Sara to find the answer she was looking for.

"I did not feel like I was being tested like Job was, but I realized I was being tested. God used a bad situation to help me advance in my spiritual development. He did not cause my son's injury nor did He allow Satan to injure my son to test me. The injury, the surgery, and the worry about AIDS were just one of those things that happens in life."

Events happen to everyone. Sometimes a bad situation is brought on by actions of another person. And sometimes a bad situation just happens. We are not always the creators of bad events in our lives. Sometimes an accident is just that, an accident.

At times like this we wonder where God is and He seems to be turning His back on us. As a result, we may turn our backs on Him or we might search for an answer elsewhere.

I AM often uses events in our lives to make us stretch and grow. These events are turned into a learning experience which will help us mature.

"The growth experienced from this situation was painful. But I guess any lesson worth learning has to hurt at times to be learned and remembered," Sara said. "I had become too comfortable and somewhat complacent in my relationship with our Supreme Being. I had stopped growing in my relationship with our Absolute Creator Being. I had even become a little smug."

Sara realized He did not cause the bad turn in events, but used them to help her learn a lesson in relationships. To have a relationship with someone you have to be engaged in interacting with them. Communication is a two-sided coin. It takes both individuals involved to be committed in conveying their thoughts and desires to each other.

"Any relationship worth having has to be nurtured. It does not matter if it is a friendship or marriage. The same is true with Source.

"I had stopped working to develop a relationship with God. I took my relationship with Father for granted. He had been doing His part, but I was not doing mine," Sara admitted.

Sara began to rebuild her relationship with I AM. How did she do it?

Confession helps to cleanse the soul. It also helped to cleanse the deep wound caused by neglect. This neglected wound was not only in Sara, but in her relationship with God.

"Asking for forgiveness was not hard for me to do," Sara said sharing her thoughts. "To admit I had been forgiven was not as easy."

Most people find it difficult to accept forgiveness. We want to keep the burden of our sin, even though our Father has forgiven us. It is within human nature to be the martyr, so we do not have to take responsibility for our actions.

"Moving ahead was my next step. I had learned from the situation and I now had to put it behind me. Dwelling on past mistakes only hinders the future."

When we are not able to feel or hear the Almighty speaking to us, we have to be careful to not fall into the trap of feeling abandoned. This trap can have devastating consequences by isolating us from our Source of Existence and our lifeline.

Fear of loneliness or autophobia is defined as an anxiety disorder which is characterized by an acute fear of being alone or isolated. It is backed with the fear of having to deal with the difficulties of life all by yourself.

Some of the issues related to feelings of abandonment are:

1. One can have issues with feelings of chronic insecurities
2. You may find yourself reenacting the traumatic event that caused the feeling of abandonment
3. Feeling unworthy and like you have been "thrown away"
4. Being overly sensitive in emotional responses to personal interactions
5. Difficulty in trusting people
6. Mood swings of depression and anxiety
7. Self-sabotaging in old and new relationships

A person who has experienced abandonment may be more likely to have long-term mental health issues. These are often based on the fear that abandonment will recur. These behaviors can alienate potential intimate partners and friends. Abandonment issues are probably one of the single most common causes of unhealthy relationships and breakups. How can we overcome fears of being left behind?

1. Stop beating yourself up. Fear of abandonment is involuntary. You did not cause it. It is the result of someone else's actions.
2. Accept this fear as part of being human. Do not judge yourself as being weak or unworthy. Cut yourself some slack and show yourself some compassion.
3. Choose to stop blaming your insecurity on other people.
4. This means taking full responsibility when your fear emerges its ugly head rather than expecting someone else to "fix it." Use the feeling of abandonment as an opportunity to develop your own sense of emotional self-reliance.
5. Approach other people with self-confidence springing forth from self-responsibility.
6. This does not just magically happen, but by becoming actively engaged in your own abandonment recovery you have taken a step forward in your emotional maturity. The reality is that, it is your responsibility to make you feel secure. The path to emotional security may take some time to walk, but as one travels this road, continue to put one foot in front of the other.
7. When you catch yourself once again looking to other people for reassurance, redirect your thoughts and get back on your own path. You are responsible for your own well-being, no one else is. Wholeness comes from within us, not from outside sources.
8. Remember that fear of abandonment is just that, a fear and it is not based in today's reality.
9. Stay calm and have realistic expectations of yourself and others.
10. Be honest with yourself and do not try to hide your feelings. See your emotions for what they are and do not exaggerate the depths of your poignant realizations.
11. Be patient, it is a learning process to accept your feelings of being left behind and realizing that you can overcome them.

12. Be in the moment now and know that you are the one who can empower your own destination.
13. Be honest with people and make your feelings known. By being authentic with others you are building emotional security.
14. By taking these steps you have empowered yourself in your road to recovery.

At times, there may be an exaggerated or irrational fear of being egotistical or being by oneself. Autophobia is an irrational fear of being egotistical or being alone.

It can cause:

~ feeling of panic,
~ feeling of terror,
~ feeling of dread, and
~ rapid heartbeat,

Why is it that we fear being alone? What is the illusion that we need to see past when it comes to being alone?

We're born alone, we live alone, we die alone. Only through our love and friendship can we create the illusion for the moment that we're not alone."

—ORSON WELLES

Orson Welles said it best in the above quote about being alone. However, this is an illusion, aloneness is part of the lie of separation from God. We are not separated from God and as a result, we are not alone.

In our self-deception of being alone, we feel isolated and vulnerable. We have been taught from the day of our birth the lie of being separated and alone. We have been conditioned to believe that we are not only separated, but we are also isolated from those around us. As humans, we have the need to be connected to or to be aware that we are a part of the greater continuum. We have the longing to feel that we belong to the larger community of people. We are taught that we are not good enough and that we have to strive to be smarter, kinder, stronger than others, and we have to work harder to earn love. In reality, we can't earn love, we are gifted love from the heart of the Eternal Light and from those individuals who care about our welfare.

Competition is learned at an early age to try to overcome the feelings of separation and isolation. We take on different roles as a person to compensate for our loneliness. But, in doing so, we lose who we really are, we lose the true essence of our soul. If we do not take the time to get to know ourselves, we will never be able to really get to know others. All of our relationships with others will be superficial.

Isolation's siblings are anger, frustration, mistrust, and jealousy. Paranoia leads us deeper into aloneness. The mind spins stories of suspicion of those around us causing us to expand the illusion of being alone. We become even more disconnected from our community and from our Creator.

God is with us, even when we think He's not. His silence is a tool He uses to help us grow. Why God chooses to be silent during difficult times is something we have to learn. There are several reasons why He chooses to be silent. And even though we may never really know why, we must realize, I AM is indeed there. He is there especially in the silence. Maybe, we are just too distracted with what is going on around us to actually hear Jehovah as He whispers in our ear. Maybe, He just wants us to be silent so He can feel our presence as we feel His.

When we study the Bible, we find it hard to relate to the world Jesus lived in. The world we live in is so distant from the things we read about in biblical history. God spoke to individuals in a more tangible way and those times seemed thrilling and glorious. We feel excluded from this intimacy He had with our distant ancestors. We feel considerably depressed and disillusioned.

How can we overcome the remoteness we feel from the disconnection of biblical experiences with Yahweh? The sense of remoteness is an illusion which comes from seeking this link between us and various Bible characters. The link between them and us is not found in times or ways of living. The connection is God Himself. The Creator with whom our ancestors had to deal with is the same Creator Source we must deal with. The basic character of I AM THAT I AM, I WILL BE WHO I WILL BE does not change.

He exists forever. He may grow older from our point of view because of our lack of understanding about time and He may expand as the Universe expands. But, He does not gain new powers, nor does He lose those that He has. He does not mature or develop. Father God cannot change for the better, He is already perfect. Because He is perfect, He cannot change for the worse. Nothing can alter the character of God.

In Exodus 3, God announces His name to Moses by saying, "I AM THAT I AM" (verse 14 NIV)—"Yahweh" (Jehovah, "the Lord") is, in effect, a shorter version (verse 15 NIV). This name is not a description of God, it's a declaration of His self-existence. It is a reminder to mankind that He has life in Him-self, and that what He is now, He always will be.

"I don't want your sacrifices—I want your love; I don't want your offerings—I want you to know me," God says through Hosea (6:6 NIV).

Knowing God creates a relationship between Him and us. We are acquainted with the Bible and Christian truths, but sometimes it does not mean much to us. But then, one day, we wake up to the fact that God is actually speaking to us through the biblical messages. We listen. We find ourselves brought very low; for Yahweh tells us about sin, guilt, weakness, and blindness. He tells us to cry out for forgiveness. But, there is more. We come to realize as we listen that God is actually opening His heart to us. He is actually making friends with us and making us a colleague. It is a startling thing, but we have now entered into a relationship with God. We entered as just a struggling human being and we were elevated to the position of a personal friend. We have gone from being a slave to the world, to a position of trust in the service of God.

The *first step* involved in knowing our Creator is listening to His word and receiving it as the Holy Spirit interprets it to us. Then we must apply it to ourselves.

Second, we must learn about Father's nature and character. These are revealed to us through His words and works. Father tells us a great deal in the creation of this world and the beauty surrounding us if only we will just look around us and see the wonders of His creation in nature. We can hear His voice in the wind as it gently blows through the leaves in the trees. We can hear His song in the music of the birds chirping and whistling their songs of joy and in the bubbling of the brook as the water meanders over the rocks. We can feel His power as the water cascades and thunders over the magnificent waterfalls. We can see Him as He commands the oceans to rise up into mighty waves. We can see His beauty in the sunrise as the light of day approaches with new blessings; and in the sunset when the light in the heavens turns into colors of shades of red, yellow, blue, and pink as the sun slowly disappears below the horizon.

Third, we accept His invitation and do what He commands. When God commands us, He is not dominating us or controlling us, but He is bringing order and structure into our world. He is guiding us into the mastery of our perception and helping us to drop the illusion of separateness. He is showing us that even in the mist of chaos, there is order.

Fourth, we recognize and rejoice in the love that He has shown us as we approach Him. He then draws us into this divine fellowship.

Knowing the Almighty Author of this world is a matter of personal dealing, just as it is with all direct acquaintances with personal relationships. Knowing God is more than knowing about Him. It is dealing with Him as He opens up to us. It is being dealt with by Him as He begins to know us.

A Bible reader and sermon listener who is full of the Holy Spirit will develop a far deeper relationship with God than the more learned man who is content with being theologically correct. Wasn't this the biggest roadblock, the greater problem for the Pharisees? The laws and keeping the laws took place over knowing God and being known by Him. God did not put the obstacles before the Pharisees, they did with their smugness and rituals. They knew a great deal about God, but they did not have intimate knowledge of Him. They did not have a personal connection to Our Father.

Knowing God, our Creator, is also a matter of personal involvement. To get to know another person, we have to commit ourselves to being in their company and learning of their interest. We have to identify with their concerns. Without this, the relationship will be superficial. Friends communicate with each other all the time. They share attitudes toward each other and toward everything else that is of common interest. They feel for one another, as well as think of one another. They nurture the friendship connection. This essential aspect of the knowledge which friends have of each other is the same principle in developing knowledge of God.

Knowing Him is an emotional and spiritual relationship as well as an intellectual one. It could not develop into a deep relationship if it were not.

Knowing Creator God is also a matter of choice and grace. The initiative throughout the relationship is from Creator. We do not make friends with Source; He makes friends with us. He brings us to know Him by making His love known to us.

"I have loved you, O my people, with an everlasting love; with lovingkindness I have drawn you to me," God tells us in Jeremiah 31:3 NIV.

In seeking a connection with All-That-There-Is, we are asking to have all veils of deception removed from our physical, psychological, spiritual, and emotional lives. Once these illusions are removed, we awaken to an internal voice of authority which calls us to turn away from external influences in our lives. As we shift from religion to spirituality, we gain access to universal truths.

Once we are open to universal truths, we may find ourselves in a spiritual crisis. This crisis can begin with an awareness of an absence of meaning and purpose in our life as we once knew it. We feel a deeper longing that is not satisfied by our present status in the community or in intimate relationships. We find that there is an unquenchable thirst as we begin to drink in the knowledge and love of our Maker.

Once we are open to universal truths, we may find ourselves in a spiritual crisis. This crisis can begin with an awareness of an absence of meaning and purpose in our life as we once knew it. We feel a deeper longing that is not satisfied by our present status in the community or in intimate relationships. We find that there is an unquenchable thirst as we begin to drink in the knowledge and love of our Maker.

The next sign we may have an awareness of is the need to experience a devotion to someone or something greater than oneself. We will feel the need to be connected to Providence in a new way. You may feel Him urging you to connect on a deeper spiritual level. Going within oneself is unsettling. We have to step out from behind the mirrors of false reflection that we have built around ourselves. It will be necessary for one to step into the clear light and see past the illusion of who we project outward into the world. You will have to come face to face with who you really are and learn to love your inner spirit.

There is a need to be devoted to a higher power than what one sees here on earth. Our devotions to other people and things are not fulfilling. There is the urge to be connected to a power beyond what we have known. We seek out our connection to the path where our divine home of the Everlasting Love resides, the only true source of who we are.

Oftentimes in a spiritual crises, one comes into conflict with the dominant worldview, and as a result we begin to feel alienated and isolated. It is necessary to have a supportive network in place to help us through the crisis so we may reach a transformative resolution. It is possible after undergoing a spiritual crisis to emerge on the other side with new insights, to develop new meanings, and to have a renewed sense of purpose. As you emerge from this crisis, you will find that you have a new found strength that has surfaced from the deep caverns within your soul. We find a strength that will keep us connected to the source of Everlasting Life.

Each of us has to have a focused purpose in life, otherwise we fall prey to unfounded fears, petty worries, imagined troubles, and feeling sorry for ourselves. This can lead to failure, sadness, and a sense of loss. This weakness cannot endure in a powerful universe that is always expanding and evolving.

Strong individuals will have a legitimate purpose in life and they will set out to obtain this goal. This purpose should be the main thought we have foremost in our mind as we go about our daily task. It may take form as a spiritual idea or a personal object, according to our needs at the time, but whatever the need is we have to steadily keep this thought in the center of our mind to move it forward into our known reality.

Doubt and fear will defeat our goals if they creep in and are allowed to remain. All that is achieved and all that is failed to be achieved is the direct result of our own thoughts. As you continue to think, there you will remain. Once a desire is identified, it can be obtained. When it is taken to the heights of aspiration, it is achieved. The seeds of our dreams then bear the fruit of truth.

In all human affairs there is an effort, and with the effort there are results. Chance has no place in forming the actuality of your world. You may find that you have an intense, burning desire within your heart that propels you forward. This is the beginning of all successful adventures. In every great passion, there is a desire that is so concentrated, that the intention will spring forward with the force of new life emerging from the barren soil of lifelessness. As the soul interprets all that we believe, think, feel, and accepts as being true, our present level of awareness will come into a clear, focused vision for you to see it unfolding into the beauty that God has intended for you to live.

After this effort has been set in motion, cultivate a physical immobility and put your efforts to sleep. This state of stillness brings with it an increased power of concentration. You can reach this state of stillness through meditation or self-hypnosis.

The seeds of your desires have now been planted in the subconscious mind for them to bloom into a desire of beauty. By seeing this fertile garden of desire in your mind and seeing it as already achieved, it will be seen in this lifetime of your creation.

Pray to the Angel of Enlightenment for understanding in any given situation. Enlightenment is a state of being, the aha moment. Enlightenment may seem elusive at times, but it is an ongoing learning process. Our outlook changes as we mature and have better understanding of the Truth we are seeking.

The Angel of Enlightenment serves as a light in the darkness of unknowingness. This light shines and sounds as a beacon to guide us to the truth we are searching for. This wonderful angelic guide gently leads us toward that which is true or in accordance with the reality of our life.

God's love is everlasting and He is unchanging, unwavering in his love for us. But man has great difficulty in being like the Creator of Life. Our love is not always everlasting and we are always changing. We are fickle beings. Because we are always changing, conflicts will arise. And since we are not as loving as we should be, forgiveness becomes a problem for some of us.

We become obsessed with our revenge and anger. When we find ourselves in this state, we are in great danger of losing our soul, of losing our very identity.

PRAYER

I take a moment to align myself with the Angel of Enlightenment and with my guardian angel. I ask for the Angel of Enlightenment to assist me in my transformation from ignorance into the knowledge of the truth that surrounds me. I pray that my eyes are opened so that I might clearly see the honesty that is before me. As I rise to a higher level of awareness, I am forever changed into a child of God who is blessed with the clarity that Father wants me to see in all situations.

I thank the Angel of Enlightenment and my guardian angel for their support and loving care while I learn to see the truth in all things. I have profound gratefulness for your blessings that you have given to me.

How can He forgive us when we cannot forgive those who have hurt us? We have cut ourselves off from God when we will not forgive others. How do we break the bonds of anger and revenge? How do we forgive?

7

Letting Go of Self-Blame

"I felt like it was my fault that my son was in trouble," Jason said. "I felt like I was a failure as a dad. I tried to be the best dad I could be for my children when my ex-wife left. I devoted all my time to taking care of my children and making sure I was giving them all my attention. I basically put my personal life on hold, so I could focus on my children and their needs. I do not know where I went wrong. But my son is always in trouble at school, he is on the verge of being expelled permanently, and now he is involved in stealing and dealing drugs. I fear that the violence of this lifestyle will catch up with him."

"My daughter started smoking at the age of nine. Now, here we are and she is in the hospital at the age of twelve with genital warts," Andy said. "It has been hard since her mother died. Allison was six when her mother died and I have done all I can to be a good father, but she just will not listen. We have gone to counseling. But she will not listen to the counselor. She has been on probation by the court system for skipping school. I do not know what else I can do."

"I'm a pediatrician, can you imagine my outrage when I learned that my sixteen-year-old son was selling drugs at school? I did not act very fatherly when I went to the police station the night my son was arrested. The police had to pull me off of my son, as I was yelling at him. I yelled at him, saying, 'You are selling drugs to these kids and I am in the emergency room trying to save their lives!'" Dr. Jim related.

It is easy to feel like a failure especially when it comes to rearing children. As a parent, we try to teach our children right from wrong, to give them all the support that we can, and still our child chooses the path of destruction. What did we do wrong? What could we have done to change the outcome? We blame ourselves, self-blame becomes our badge of failure. Our own Scarlet Letter to be worn. Why is it so hard for us to realize that our children are individuals and the choices they make are their responsibility? Why do we bash ourselves for our children's bad decisions?

We do not want to admit to ourselves that our children want to live a lifestyle we consider to be dangerous or at the very least poor judgement. We do not want to admit that our son or daughter will make their own choices in spite of what we are trying to do to help them. Oftentimes, they turn their backs on the very help they are offered so they can make better life choices. Or, so they think, they know better than we do. They do not need or want our advice.

Self-blame is considered one of the most abusive emotions we can place on ourselves. Why is it that we refuse to extend lovingkindness to ourselves? We are not perfect and we fail to recognize our own humanity. We, as parents, feel that we have the need to be right all the time, especially when it comes to our children. We want to give our children the best advice we can and we do not want to make a mistake in guiding our children.

Self-blame can keep us stuck in the muck and gooeyness on the shadow side of our emotions. Why is it so hard for us to have self-acceptance? Why is it easier for us to recognize the human imperfection in ourselves before we can see it in others? We are not perfect and we are not going to be right every time. We create an opportunity for learning, self-discovery, and personal growth for others, but not for ourselves. Why is that?

What happens to our physical and psychological health when we nurture chronic stress? Our mind and body are inseparably linked. And the intercommunication between mind and body can produce physical changes that are lasting. Our brain becomes aware of a stressor and a physical reaction is triggered. This reaction can lead to a backlash of emotional responses. This can cause mental and physical damage to the individual. Some problems such as headaches, muscle tension, and muscle pain are often directly caused by the body's response to stress. Other health issues such as diverticulitis, arthritis, insomnia, hypertension, diabetes, and heart disease to name a few, can be exacerbated due to persistent stress. If chronic stress is not alleviated irreversible damage can be done to the body causing life-threatening situations such as heart attack or stroke.

We are not going to get it right every time, in every situation or in every relationship. We have to release self-blame, especially in situations where other people are responsible for their own actions.

The first step in releasing self-blame is recognizing responsibility, who owns the decision and where does the ownership lie? Have we done all we could do in the situation to be honest? If so, then, when things go wrong it will be clear where our responsibility lies.

The second step is to take responsibility or letting the other person take responsibility for their own actions in the situation.

If you are prone to self-blame, follow these tips:

~ Pay attention to your thoughts and emotions. Self-blame has a lot more power when it happens automatically. Once you realize you are doing it, you can take control of it. Practice Mindful Thought, focus on the here and now. Focus on what is happening in the current moment.

~ Identify the source of the self-blame. What problem are you blaming yourself for having?

~ Look for the root cause of the problem. Could it possibly have been seeded in your childhood? Could you have grown up with some form of childhood emotional neglect?

~ Have compassion for yourself. It will free you to address the true problem at hand. (7) (8)

What steps can we take to be kinder to ourselves?

~ Set attainable and realistic goals. Do you have clear-sighted expectations? Have you considered the other person's desires and their free will?

~ Do not accept the negative, unjustified self-criticism. It has no useful benefit and it becomes a death trap preventing you in moving forward.

~ Be your own best friend. Jesus told us to love ourselves as we love others. He did not tell us to love others instead of ourselves.

~ Find a way to destress. Take a walk, a relaxing bath, meditation, reconnect with nature, pray.

~ Spend time every week on a self-improvement project. Expand your horizons.

~ Declare that you are going to be kinder to yourself and work toward that goal. (7) (8)

As a parent, we want the best for our children, but at some point we have to learn to let go and realize that our child is an individual. As an individual, this child has free will and we cannot take their free will away from them. We can't prevent our offspring from making mistakes, even dangerous mistakes. It is hard for us as parents when we see our adolescent walking down a destructive path to sit back and do nothing. But, we have to realize at some point that, as an individual, this human being will make their own choices and there is nothing that we can do to prevent them from making a destructive choice.

Some individuals have to learn life's lessons the hard way. For some, this is the only way they are able to learn the lessons of life. It is hard as a parent to see our son or daughter walk down a destructive path. In reality, we do not always have a choice in the matter. This child of ours has free will and is determined to do things their own way. Often our strong-willed, hardheaded adolescent will do just the opposite of what we tell them just to prove we do not have control over them.

In those situations, self-blame only gets in the way, it becomes a hindrance. If we take on self-blame, then we are not being realistic about what is going in our life or the life of our child or teenager or young adult. We are not able to think clearly. We are not allowing this individual to learn to take responsibility for their own actions. We are, in fact, teaching them to lay blame on others for their actions. We are setting our children up for failure if we do not make them take responsibility for their own decisions, their own actions. Sometimes the hardest part of being a parent is letting our children fail, to let them trip and fall flat on their faces. Without failure, they do not grow or learn life's valuable lessons. Without growth, they are never able to become self-reliant adults. They do not know what it is to be responsible for their own actions and they do not recognize the damage they do to others. They become narrow-sighted and blind to life's lessons.

As hard as it is to let a youngster fail, to fall flat on their face, we become part of the problem instead of part of the solution if we continue to interfere. If we persist in interfering with our child's learning experience, then we have turned that individual into an emotionally damaged person. Self-blame has no upside when we have not wronged another. We are no longer setting an example on how to be a responsible adult, but we are teaching our children how to avoid responsibility for their own actions.

So, as a parent, how do we move past self-blame? How do we let go of our children and let them learn their life's lessons? Why do teenagers chose crime?

What Children/Teenagers Learn From Failing:

~ Responsibility

Responsibility is the act of doing what is right when there is no authoritative person around to make one choose the right course of action. In other words, it is doing the right thing when no one is looking. Internal motivation develops when teens are made to be accountable for their actions. Making teenagers accountable when they make a mistake will cause them a degree of discomfort, and discomfort can be one of life's biggest motivators. This uneasiness teaches them compassion for others and for themselves.

~ Coping Skills

By allowing teenagers the chance to experience failure and difficulty, you enable them to develop important coping skills, which they will call upon throughout their lifetime. They will learn to think outside of the box and become more creative.

~ Learn To Adapt

In order to live a full life we all need to learn how to change and adjust when things do not go as planned. The ability to adjust, improvise, reprioritize, compromise, and to change is vital in a world that is forever changing. We must learn to be flexible in different situations. If our child can't learn to adapt to the ever-changing world in which we live, they will be crippled and will always have problems in dealing with day to day life. They will struggle with the simplest aspects of life without coping skills.

~ Learn Not to Fear Failure

Giving children and young adults the freedom to fall short and to make mistakes allows them to explore their own creativity, to learn real-life lessons, and to develop a deeper understanding of the world. When your child falls flat on their face, they learn who they are and where their place is in the overall scheme of things. It helps them learn about interactions with the people they will come into contact with.

~ Learn to Deal With Disappointment

Life is full of disappointments. Prepare your child for independence by not shielding them from setbacks and failures, but allowing them to be exposed to the reality that things do not always turn out as they planned. Life is hard. Life situations can be extremely difficult and painful at times and if we, as parents, are always trying to "fix" our offspring's mistakes, we are also teaching them that they are not competent to take care of their own lives and walk their own path.

~ Learn Not to Feel Entitled

When we shield our son or daughter from disappointment or failure, they form a sense of entitlement. They believe they deserve success or happiness simply because they are who they are. When our adolescent accepts responsibility for failure, they learn to solve problems by acknowledging and dealing with them rather than blaming others or using manipulation to get their own way. We do not get a trophy for just "showing up" in life. There are winners and losers in life. That is the way of the world.

As a parent, there will come a point in time when we just have to let go, we have to learn that our child's choices are theirs alone. We are not to take on self-blame when our children are given the tools to live a productive life and they chose to ignore or reject making productive choices. As our young adult children mature, we have to accept that they may make the decision to do what society considers to be out of the norm or breaking the law in spite of our teaching them the expectations of harmonious living.

Would you take on the self-blame for your cousin's mistakes? Of course not. It really is not any different with your children. Our individual children have free will and they will exercise this free will whether or not we like it. God allows us to exercise our free will even if it is for our own determent. If Father knows that at times we have to fail in order to grow and learn life's lessons, then who are we to refuse to allow our children the opportunity to learn and grow from their mistakes?

Here are a few tips when you find yourself or others blaming you for your child's behavior:

1. Keep the focus where it belongs, on your child's behavior. Their behavior is just that, theirs.

2. Learn to balance your parental responsibility with your child's accountability. Accept responsibility for what you feel is your job as a parent and allow your child to accept responsibility for his own choices. Your ultimate goal is to raise a child who will be able to function responsibly in the adult world. You can't do that if you continue to interfere in the process.

3. Keep the Big Picture in mind. You guided your son or daughter, cared for them and prepared them for the Real

World. He or she is here to make this life their own, to learn and to grow. Blaming yourself for their behavior does not help in those life tasks. It stunts the young adult's ability to figure out for themselves what they are comfortable with if they are not allowed to make their own choices. Unless they are encouraged to decide what decisions feel good and right to him or her, this individual will be handicapped and incapable of making choices. They will have problems in deciding what kind of person they are going to be when they become adults.

4. Develop a Culture of Accountability that the child must live within. Define the parameters that you expect your son or daughter to live within. Accountability starts at home. When we blame ourselves for our teenagers struggles, it leads to guilt and shame. Shame is a "Parenting Immobilizer": it renders us ineffective when it comes to responding to our offspring. This can lead to us avoiding holding our child accountable for their own actions. If you feel guilty or ashamed for things you have done as a parent, take accountability and move forward. If you hold your child accountable for their own actions, they will be on the path to becoming a responsible, well–adjusted adult. (10)

Let's face it, parenting is the hardest job you will do in this lifetime. Sometimes, parenting is the worst life experience we can have. Life is messy. Children do not come with instruction manuals. Parenting is a learning process. Often we learn "by the seat of our pants." We will make mistakes, every parent does. There will be incidents when no matter how loving, how understanding, how self-sacrificing you are as a parent, your son or daughter will rip your heart out, tear it into shreds, and stomp on it. In some cases, we may be judged by our child's actions, especially if that individual child has committed an offense that society has deemed as inexcusable. It seems as though there are more of these issues arising in our society today. Violence is becoming more prevalent with mass murders being committed by teenagers.

Teen violence refers to harmful behaviors that can start early and continue into young adulthood. The young person can be a victim, an offender, or a witness to the violence. Violent acts can include: bullying, fighting, including punching, kicking, slapping, or hitting. Also, violent acts include the use of weapons such as guns or knives.

The Center for Disease Control (CDC) provides these 2010 statistics on teen violence regarding violent crimes:

- ~ 4,828 young people, ages 10–24, were victims of homicide. An average of 13 each day.
- ~ 82.8 percent of youth homicides were committed with a firearm.
- ~ Juveniles under 18 accounted for 13.7 percent of all violent crime arrests and 22.5% of all property crime arrests.
- ~ 784 juveniles were arrested for murder.
- ~ 2,198 juveniles were arrested for forcible rape.
- ~ 35,001 juveniles were arrested for aggravated assault.

What makes teenagers commit violent acts? Why does it seem to be more prevalent now than in past years? It would take a separate book just to examine these two questions, but I do want to take a brief look at some of the causes of teen violence.

The frontal lobe of teenagers which is the part of the brain that is important in higher functioning, decision making, and controlling impulses, and their connections to other parts of the brain do not mature until around the age of twenty-five. It seems that the myelin in the brain of a teenager is underdeveloped. The myelin is the connective tissue which helps brain signals flow freely and efficiently between the frontal lobes and the rest of the brain. This underdevelopment contributes to the signals moving much more slowly in undeveloped brains.

Hasn't this always been the way the brain has developed? So, why does it seem that teen violence is more prominent today than in past generations?

The reasons are vast and more complicated than what this book will cover, but children are exposed to more violent movies, television shows, games, and experiences in day-to-day living than children in past generations. They become desensitized to violence when they are exposed to such behavior. It does not matter if they are seeing it in a television show, movie, or video game. Constant exposure to aggression is in some ways turning horrible events into the norm. We are no longer shocked at such behavior when we are being bombarded by it daily.

With both parents working in most households, this means that teens have more unsupervised time either alone or with peers who are not necessarily a good influence. There is in some cases a lack of attachment to the parents since the parents are away from the home working long hours.

Teens growing up in homes with a lower income and less education are more likely to engage in violent behavior. Parents who abuse drugs or alcohol also increase a teen's risk of behaving violently.

Stressful family environments, such as a lack of a father in the home to provide male guidance, conflict in the home between family members, or lack of parental role modeling of appropriate behavior contribute to a teen's sense of worthlessness which can lead to violent behavior. Lack of direction for both the teens and parents make modern living more difficult. This being said, these factors make parenting harder than in previous years.

In the above section, we have looked at how destructive self-blame is and you have been given the tools to work through this unjustified torture that you have placed on yourself. But, in reality, there are those of you out there who will continue to self-blame for your child's actions in spite of what you know to be true.

You are the people I am talking with now. You think you show compassion to others. You most certainly will show compassion to your child whether or not this individual turns their life around or not.

My question to you is: Why are you not showing this same compassion to yourself? You are a child of God, He loves you and does not hold you to blame for others misdeeds. Why are you continuing to hold yourself responsible for the choices your young adult insists on making?

I encourage you to seek professional help if you are not able to break this vicious cycle you find yourself in. If you can't show compassion for yourself, then you will not be able to show true compassion for anyone else.

How can Father forgive you when you can't forgive yourself? He does not hold us guilty for the "sins of our children" when we have taken the appropriate steps to teach them right from wrong. We do not take on the "sins of the father" nor should we take on the "sins of the children."

PRAYER

I call on the Angel of Compassion and my guardian angel to help me show compassion to myself as Father God has shown compassion to me. Help me to see beyond the veil of self-blame. Help me to see self-blame for what it is, destructive and binding me into a belief that is false.

I call on Spirit Most High to lift the veil that obstructs my true vision. Spirit Most High, you are the living word of Compassion. Show me how to have compassion for myself. Show me how to extend empathy to myself and to let go of the self-blame I have imposed on myself.

I thank the Angel of Compassion and my guardian angel for helping me move beyond self-blame and to restore my true sense of value to myself.

8

From the Dark Abyss of Depression into the Light of Love

" I really just do not want to be here anymore. I just do not care if I live or die. I have no plans to harm myself and I would not do that to my family, but I would not be upset if I died either."

"Why am I alive? It should have been me who died and not my friend."

I have heard these statements or other similar statements made throughout the course of my career in the medical field too many times to count.

It is reported that an estimated sixteen million American adults, almost 7 percent of the population, have had at least one major depressive episode in the past year. People of all ages and all racial, ethnic, and socioeconomic backgrounds experience depression, but it does affect some groups more than others.

About 5 percent of children and adolescents in the general population suffer from depression at any given point in time. Children under stress, who experience loss, or who have attention, learning, conduct, or anxiety disorders are at a higher risk for depression. Depression also tends to run in families.

A new study finds that African Americans and Latinos are significantly more likely to experience serious depression than whites.

Why is depression so prevalent in our society? Is there a common denominator contributing to the numbers of people suffering from depression? Is there more depression in current day society than in past generations? If so, why? What are the symptoms of depression? What are the causes of depression? How does one deal with depression? Can one overcome depression?

So, are more people depressed today, than say, fifty years ago? The exact number varies from study to study, so it is unclear by how much the rate of depression has increased. But, that depression has become more common, that seems certain. Or is it? Could it be that we have better diagnostic tools? Are we better at identifying and reporting the statistics of individuals who are depressed?

Past generations lived through World War I and World War II, they lived through the great depression and experienced the horrors of those times. They experienced the fear of not having enough food to feed their families during the years of drought and when crops failed during the early twentieth century. They were considered to be survivors of perilous times. This generation was known as being "tough as old boots." Millions of people were fighting for basic necessities of food, water, and shelter just to live. It certainly was not an easy time in history.

Current society has its challenges as well. Our stress is of a different nature. Five of the top stressors in current day society are listed as death of a loved one, divorce, moving, major illness, and loss of a job.

Are not today's stressors just as stressful as early twentieth-century society? Today's society has seen its hardships with military conflicts and homelessness as well. So, what is the difference?

More than fifty years ago, people were taught to "buck up" and deal with it and get on with life. Men were taught to hold in their feelings and be strong. Real men did not cry, at least not in front of other people.

In today's society, everyone talks about their feelings. Children get trophies for just showing up for a sports event, after all, we do not want anyone to have their feelings hurt. Our lifestyle is easier than past generations, we have more efficient heating and cooling, food is plentiful, transportation is readily available, and medical treatment is easy to come by.

Sadly, mental health was not well understood in the late nineteenth and early twentieth centuries. The prevailing view at the time was one of institutionalization. People with learning disabilities or mental health conditions found themselves sent to asylums and other similar institutions, to live apart from the rest of society. These institutions were thought of as places of treatment, where people could be given specialized care, but they were also places of segregation. We did not want to see the defective individuals of our communities. It frightened us and we did not know what to do with them or how to act around them.

Fortunately attitudes have evolved to some extent. Mental health has been taken out of the back of the closet and has been brought out into the open. Let's take a look at the definition of depression.

Medical depression is defined as an illness that involves the body, mood, and thoughts and that affects the way a person eats, sleeps, feels about himself or herself, and thinks about things.

Symptoms are identified as:

~ changes in sleep,
~ changes in appetite,

~ lack of concentration,
~ loss of energy,
~ lack of interest in activities,
~ hopelessness or guilty thoughts,
~ changes in movement (less activity or agitation),
~ physical aches and pains, and
~ suicidal thoughts,

Depression is not:

~ something you can 'snap out of,'
~ a sign of weakness,
~ something that everyone experiences, or
~ something that lasts forever

Here is a list of some of the many causes of depression:

~ Trauma, especially experienced at an early age, can cause long-term changes in how the brain responds to fear and stress. These changes may lead to depression.
~ Genetics: Mood disorders, such as depression, tend to run in families.
~ Life circumstances: Marital status, relationship changes, financial standing, and where a person lives can influence whether a person develops depression or not. Stressors are just as great in each step of the ladder.
~ Brain changes: Imaging studies have shown that the frontal lobe of the brain becomes less active when a person is depressed. Depression is also associated with changes in how the pituitary gland and hypothalamus respond to hormone stimulation.
~ Other medical conditions: People who are depressed have a history of sleep disturbances, medical illness, chronic pain, anxiety, and attention-deficit hyperactivity disorder

(ADHD). They are more likely to develop chronic depression that will be more difficult to break the chemical cycle in the brain. Some medical syndromes (like hypothyroidism) can mimic depressive disorder. Many medications can also cause symptoms of depression.

~ Drug and alcohol abuse: Approximately 30 percent of people with substance abuse problems also have depression. This requires coordinated treatment for both conditions, as alcohol can worsen symptoms. (14)

To be diagnosed with a depressive disorder, a person must have experienced a depressive episode lasting longer than two weeks. The symptoms of a depressive episode include:

~ loss of interest or loss of pleasure in all activities,
~ change in appetite or weight,
~ sleep disturbances,
~ feeling agitated or feeling slowed down,
~ fatigue,
~ feelings of low self-worth, guilt, or shortcomings,
~ difficulty concentrating or making decisions; and
~ suicidal thoughts or intentions

For chronic depression treatment can include:

~ psychotherapy including cognitive behavioral therapy, family-focused therapy, and interpersonal therapy
~ medications such as antidepressants, mood stabilizers, and antipsychotic medications
~ exercise that can help with prevention and mild-to-moderate symptoms
~ brain stimulation therapies that can be tried if psychotherapy and/or medication are not effective. These include electroconvulsive therapy (ECT) for depressive disorder with

psychosis or repetitive transcranial magnetic stimulation (rTMS) for severe depression
~ light therapy, which uses a light box to expose a person to full spectrum light in an effort to regulate the hormone melatonin
~ alternative approaches including acupuncture, meditation, faith and nutrition that can be part of a comprehensive treatment plan, but do not have strong scientific backing (14)

According to the National Institute of Mental Health, suicide is the 10th leading cause of death in the United States. Every year 44,965 Americans die by suicide. For every suicide there are 25 others who attempted suicide. The annual cost of suicide is $69 billion.

But how can you put a price on the devastation of suicide? Children who have had a parent commit suicide are more likely to commit suicide themselves than children whose parents do not commit suicide.

An area of mental health called accidental suicide is one area that is hard to gather statistics on. Accidental suicide is defined as an individual who in a rash moment attempts to take their own life, but too late regrets their action. They realize moments before death that they really didn't want to take their own life.

The annual age-adjusted suicide rate is 13.42 per 100,000 individuals.

~ Men die by suicide 3.53 times more often than women.
~ On average, there are 123 suicides per day.
~ White males accounted for 7 of 10 suicides in 2016.
~ Firearms account for 51 percent of all suicides in 2016.
~ The rate of suicide is highest in middle age—white men in particular.

Depression is a symptom that still is not well understood. Depression is considered an emotional and mental disorder. Chronic depression often precedes the development of a physical illness such as chronic headache, stomachache, heart disease, and obesity.

Depression is also a common condition in certain diseases like Parkinson's, Dementia, and Multiple Sclerosis. People who have chronic pain often also suffer from depression.

Depression weakens the immune system causing it to plummet making the individual prone to infections and other infectious diseases. Thyroid levels can affect depression and should be checked.

Antidepressants are drugs used for the treatment of major depressive disorders and other conditions, including dysthymia, anxiety disorders, obsessive–compulsive disorder, eating disorders, chronic pain, neuropathic pain and, in some cases, dysmenorrhea, snoring, migraine, attention-deficit hyperactivity disorder (ADHD), addiction, dependence, and sleep disorders. They may be prescribed alone or in combination with other medications. Most types of antidepressants are typically safe to take, but these medications may cause increased thoughts of suicide and worsening depression.

From the metaphysical viewpoint depression is also a release of energy and the individual is not conscious of the drained energy being released from the body. Depression affects our ability to heal. The emotions of anger, bitterness, rage, and resentment interfere with healing by blocking the internal power that our body has to fight disease. Depression robs one of their internal power and energy leaving them defenseless.

Healing requires the unity of the mind, heart, and body. More often than not, it is the mind that needs to be adjusted to what we are feeling. We have to honor our emotions before we can begin the healing process. We have to listen to what our heart is telling us. What we think, we become. Pay attention to what you think.

What are some of the nonmedical tools we can use to help relieve depression? Hypnosis has become recognized as a potentially effective treatment for many individuals with depression. Some recent studies have shown that it is more effective than cognitive-behavioral therapy, which is the most common therapy approach in treating clinical depression.

Hypnosis has been used for several decades for depression. However, it has only been in recent years that hypnosis has been recognized in the medical community as a viable tool. Hypnosis for depression can identify and address the underlying cause or the root cause of the individual's symptoms. It can assist individuals in finding more effective coping skills. It can also assist people in achieving a happier mood and decrease or eliminate the pessimistic and negative thoughts that generally accompany depression.

Guided imagery is also a valuable tool to help with depression. Guided imagery is a self-help or therapeutic intervention during which a person visualizes or imagines things suggested in order to create physiological and psychological healing. It is the least expensive, safest, and often most effective way to help resolve most illnesses. With guided imagery mental pictures are created by using descriptive words that will bring images into the mind's eye. These images and thoughts are indistinguishable to your body and nervous system. Guided imagery creates a positive inner image of your body, or health status, and by working with the deeper levels of your subconscious can create positive results. Guided imagery helps to reduce stress by causing a feeling of calmness and helps enhance wellness and promotes improved health.

Here are some of the benefits of guided imagery:

1. deep relaxation of muscles and other organs
2. helps your body work with you and not against you
3. helps your body heal faster from illness or injury

4. reduces stress and anxiety
5. promotes a deeper spiritual connection
6. helps to eliminate self-destructive behaviors
7. improves sleep
8. improves communication
9. assists in having authentic relationships

While guided imagery is generally considered safe when used correctly, it is important to note that this technique should not be used as a substitute for the mental-health-professional care of depression.

Meditation is a mind/body practice that has been used for centuries for increasing calmness and physical relaxation. Meditation helps to improve psychological balance, coping with illness, and enhancing overall wellness and mental clarity. Mind and body practice focuses on the interactions among the brain, mind, body, and behavior.

~ Meditation is one of the best techniques to transform your mental well being naturally. Meditation is not only about relaxation. It will also help you to reduce and eliminate anxiety and stress. Meditation helps to remove the mental chatter from the conscious mind that is so distracting for many people. Meditation allows one to mentally clear away stressors, thoughts, and worries that need to be reconciled while in a meditative state.

~ The primary purpose of meditation is not to dissolve your anxiety, but instead, it is to help you become more centered in the present. It helps one to focus on the here and now. Focus on your breathing to help you become centered. Breathe from the diaphragm for the positive effects of deep breathing.

~ Meditation allows us to slow down, have a new perspective on the present moment, and to become more objective in our thinking. (21)

Prayer has been shown to decrease depression and anxiety. The relationship between prayer and health has been the subject of scores of double-blind studies over the past four decades. Researchers at Baylor and Harvard and many other colleges have reported that people who pray have better outcomes than people who do not pray.

Spiritual practice using prayer aims to connect the individual with God or their Higher Power. Prayer can open you to the Divine power dwelling within the self and to make you fully present to be in the here and now.

Lisa Miller, PhD, professor and director of Clinical Psychology and director of the Spirituality Mind Body Institute at Teachers College, Columbia University, demonstrated that people who placed spirituality and religion as a high priority were less likely to suffer from depression. A study, published on December 25, 2013, is the first published investigation on the neuro-correlates of the protective effect of spirituality and religion against depression. This study revealed that brain MRIs showed thicker cortices in people who placed a high importance on religion or spirituality than those who did not. The relatively thicker cortex was found in precisely the same regions of the brain that had otherwise shown thinning in people at high risk for depression. A thicker cortex indicates a smaller chance of suffering from depression, suggesting that prayer and spirituality really does reveal some very remarkable benefits to the human brain.

It has been shown that prayer has similar effects and benefits on an individual as does meditation. Prayer can improve a person's mental health, such as reducing anxiety and stress. When stress levels are reduced, lower levels of the stress hormone cortisol are noted in the body resulting in lower blood pressure, and improved immune functioning.

Here are some benefits of prayer:

~ Increased focus and attention
~ Mental clarity is noted with prayer. Prayer clears the mind of distractions and negative thoughts
~ Better control over thoughts and less intrusive thoughts
~ Guards against depression
~ Improved short-term and long-term memory
~ Decreased anxiety and fear
~ Positive thinking and better outlook on life
~ Stress reduction
~ Increases one's ability to relax and become calm
~ Promotes a restful night's sleep
~ Increases overall sense of well-being
~ Prayer builds a sense of confidence (22)

There is a correlation between an increase of alpha brain waves with prayer and mindfulness and meditation producing the ability to reduce depressive symptoms and increase creative thinking.

With prayer, mindfulness, and meditation one is able to step into a realm of spiritual protection. It is within this realm of protection that we can pour out the pain and anguish causing our soul such distress. It is within this dimensional realm that we feel the gentle embrace of Divine Love and Comfort. In this dimension of love, we are able to release some of the distress that depression has placed within our soul.

In another study, Sarah Lazar, a neuroscientist at Harvard Medical School, has studied the benefits of prayer in brain scans. She found that it greatly affected the amygdala by making this part of the brain shrink; the part that is connected to anxiety, depression, and stress. The participants who meditated or prayed were, in essence, able to better handle depression—the well-known state of mind that has been labeled the illness that engulfs America today. Depression and mental pain are one of the most common mental disorders in the U.S., according to the National Institute of Mental Health. (20)

Mindfulness is defined as paying attention to one's experience in the present moment. It involves observing thoughts and emotions from moment to moment without judging or becoming caught up in them. A study in *The Lancet* found that Mindfulness helped prevent depression recurrence as effectively as maintenance dose antidepressant medication did.

Practicing mindfulness exercises can have many positive benefits including reduced stress, anxiety, and depression. Less negative thinking and distraction. Improved mood.

Other benefits of mindfulness include:

1. An improved overall sense of well-being—by focusing on the here and now, it is easier not to get caught up in worrying about things that may or may not happen.
2. Improved physical health—mindfulness helps to reduce stress, maintain a healthier blood pressure, reduces pain, and improves sleep along with many other physical improvements.
3. Improved mental health—depression, substance abuse, eating disorders, anxiety disorders, and obsessive-compulsive disorder.

We have a number of tools in our health toolbox that we can use in combating depression. You may find it helpful to use a variety of these tools to maintain your mental and physical health. There are other tools that can be added such as physical exercise. Regular exercise may help ease depression and anxiety by:

~ releasing feel-good endorphins, natural cannabis-like brain chemicals (endogenous cannabinoids) and other natural brain chemicals that can enhance your sense of well-being

~ taking your mind off worries so you can get away from the cycle of negative thoughts that feed depression and anxiety

A healthy diet can play an important role in reduction of depression and anxiety as well as improving overall health. Fresh fruits and vegetables and plant-based foods with whole grains will give the body and mind the nutrients needed to maintain good health.

There are some foods that can contribute to depression and anxiety. These foods include sugar, artificial sweeteners, processed foods, hydrogenated oils, foods high in sodium, alcohol, and caffeine. In a study published in the journal *Diabetologia*, researchers have found that when blood glucose levels are elevated, levels of a protein that encourages the growth of neurons and synapses drops.

Artificial sweeteners found in products like diet soda blocks the production of the neurotransmitter serotonin. This can cause all manner of neurological problems including headaches, insomnia, changes in mood, and depression.

Alcohol is a depressant, and more specifically, depresses the working order of the central nervous system.

Hydrogenated oils go through a process called hydrogenation that turns vegetable oil into a more solid form, which makes it a more shelf-stable product. However, hydrogenated oil can potentially contribute to depression.

According to a 2012 study in the journal *Public Health Nutrition*, people who eat fast food are 51 percent more likely to develop depression than those who do not.

Caffeine can contribute to depression because of caffeine's disruptive effect on sleep. Coffee and black tea make it more difficult to fall asleep and to stay asleep. Sleep disturbances are connected to mood and disturbed sleep can cause serious complications with your mental state. Lack of sleep, if it goes on long enough, can cause seizures and even death in some extreme cases.

Here are foods that can help decrease depression and anxiety:

~ Whole grain is rich in magnesium, and magnesium deficiency may lead to anxiety.
~ Whole grain contains tryptophan, which becomes serotonin—a calming neurotransmitter.
~ Whole grains create healthy energy while reducing hunger—both important for anxiety.
~ Seaweed is a good alternative to whole grains for those that are gluten sensitive. Seaweed appears to have a high magnesium content, and kelp and other seaweed appear to be very high in tryptophan content.
~ Blueberries are rich in vitamins and phytonutrients (plant nutrients), and have a variety of antioxidants that are considered extremely beneficial for relieving stress.
~ Almonds are an underrated food. Almonds contain zinc, a key nutrient for maintaining a balanced mood and have both iron and healthy fats. Healthy fats are an important part of a balanced diet, and low iron levels have been known to cause brain fatigue, which can contribute to both anxiety and a lack of energy.

Maintaining a healthy diet is important for overall health and wellness. A diet rich in whole grains, vegetables, and fruits is a healthier option than eating simple carbohydrates found in processed foods. Do not skip meals. Skipping meals may result in drops in blood sugar that cause you to feel jittery, which can contribute to worsening anxiety.

I urge anyone who is struggling with depression to seek help. In some cases it may take trying different therapies, medications, and combinations of each to find an effective treatment. Do not give up! There is a light at the end of the Dark Abyss and in that light is love and joy.

Psalms 40:1–3: I waited patiently for the LORD; he inclined to me and heard my cry. He drew me up from the pit of destruction, out of the miry bog, and set my feet upon a rock, making my steps secure. He put a new song in my mouth, a song of praise to our God. Many will see and fear, and put their trust in the LORD. (NIV)

PRAYER

I call on the Angel of Desperation and my guardian angel to help me find my way out of this pit of depression. Please grab my hand firmly and pull me out of this abyss of despair. Help me to see beyond the despair and pain to see the truth. Help me to see the truth that all is not lost and that God is with me as I walk through the valley of despair.

Guide me toward the Light of Hope and into the hands of the Angel of Hope. Help me see the truth that Hope is with me always.

SERENITY PRAYER:

God Grant Me the Serenity To Accept the Things I Cannot Change;
The Courage to Change the Things I Can;
And the Wisdom to Know the Difference.

9

The Regret of Love Lost

"She's beautiful, intelligent, smart, and funny," Adam said. "I just could not take my eyes off of her when we first met. I met Annie at a coworker's retirement party. The auditorium was full of people wishing our coworker well and she was looking for a place to sit down to eat. There was an open chair next to me and Ann asked if the seat was taken. I pushed the chair back for her and told her 'no, it is not taken.' It was like we had known each other all our lives and we talked through the entire lunch. I remember thinking as she left the auditorium that I wanted to see her again."

Adam could not wait for the next day to come. Annie's office was one floor down from his office. The next day Adam had to meet with the staff on his team and as fate would have it, Annie's office was next door to the rest of his team. Adam had the perfect opportunity to stop by Annie's office to say hello. From that day forward Adam would go to Annie's office each day to talk with her. It was not long before he was meeting Annie at the end of the day to walk out with her. It was obvious to Annie that Adam wanted to ask her out, but six months later he still had not asked her out. He just could not seem to move forward. The fact that Adam was not moving forward in the relationship puzzled Ann.

What happens when we do not move forward in relationships? Especially in situations that involve the heart. Missed opportunities in love can cause the deepest, saddest regret we will ever experience.

Regret is defined as a negative conscious and emotional reaction to one's personal decision-making, a choice resulting in action or inaction. Regret is related to perceived missed opportunity or perceived remorse over something done that we wish we had not done. Its intensity varies over time after the decision or indecision, in regard to action versus in-action, and in regard to self-control at a particular point in time. The self-recrimination which comes with regret is thought to spur corrective action and adaptation. (15)

Adam had been blindsided by his intensely deep feelings for Annie. Adam was panicked by this surprised turn in events and soon he began to avoid Annie. Annie could not understand what had caused the change in Adam's behavior toward her, so, she decided the relationship had just run its course.

In the next few weeks, Annie decided to take a job in a town four hours away from Adam. Adam came to Annie's office to talk with her just before attending a "going away party" that her coworkers were having for her. On the way out of Annie's office, Annie tapped Adam on the arm and said, "If you had asked me out like you were supposed to, we could have been having a lot of fun."

Annie's comment stopped Adam dead in his tracks. That moment in time stood still as he realized that this was an opportunity lost.

Love lost is one of life's biggest and saddest regrets. Adam realized after Annie had moved that he was having thoughts about Annie and feeling overwhelmed by the coulda-shoulda-woulda of his inaction in telling Annie how he felt about her and not moving forward in the relationship. How can we deal with the regrets that just will not go away? What happens if we do not face these regrets?

The cumulative effect of living with regret can have a debilitating impact on your physical and psychological health. Some of the common symptoms of chronic regret is a feeling of helplessness, depression, lack of energy, eating disorders (i.e., either eating too much or not enough), and sleep disorders (i.e., sleeping too much or not getting enough sleep). If regret is not dealt with, it quickly becomes chronic stress which will cause other physical symptoms of hypertension, headaches, anxiety, and panic attacks among numerous other symptoms.

How do we deal with regret? What steps should we take to regain our physical and mental and emotional health?

1. Be honest with yourself about your feelings. Do not try to ignore them or indulge them. Recognize your feelings and acknowledge them, face the disappointment, feel the pain that comes with the sadness, learn from the loss, forgive yourself, and see it for what it is: life's lessons.

2. Facing your remorse involves examining what feelings you have buried under the grief or what it is covering up. Are you experiencing sorrow? Are you having anger with yourself for your actions or lack of action? Is disappointment a primary symptom? Is disillusionment with yourself holding you captive? Or is there a mixture of the above symptoms? Determine what your emotions are and be honest with yourself. You do not need to do anything. You just need to be aware of your feelings,

neither indulging nor repressing. Just experience them and see them for what they are. Be brave.

3. Learn from your experience. Think about what you could have done differently. Determine if you want to rectify the situation by reaching out to the other person involved in the situation. If you do want to correct the situation, think about the steps you need to take to make amends and move forward.

A few months later, Annie was back in town to be with her daughter who having surgery. Annie visited her former coworkers while she was in town. While Annie was waiting for one of her friends to return to the Mental Health Outpatient building where she had worked, Annie knocked on Adam's office door. Adam was surprised to see Annie and pulled her into his new office, which just now happened to be next door to her old office. Adam began to tell Annie how he felt about her and why he did not ask her out. Annie was stunned to learn that Adam had deep feelings for her. The conversation was interrupted when one of Adam's team members knocked on his office door. Annie left Adam's office in a stunned daze.

For the next few months, Adam and Annie saw each other when Annie was in town. Adam told Annie of two past relationships that were very painful for him. Adam would take one step forward, then two steps backward in trying to establish a relationship with Annie.

What happens when one becomes so stuck in fear that they cannot move forward in a relationship? What can be done to move ahead in life? Is there a name for being fearful of love?

The fear of love, or falling in love is a phobia known as Philophobia. Philophobia is an unwarranted and an irrational fear of falling in love. Occasionally, the individual does fall in love, but in most cases it causes such an intense emotional turmoil within the individual's mind that they are paralyzed and unable to move forward.

What are some of the causes of philophobia?

~ It is believed that an intensely negative love experience in the past might have triggered the reaction. Watching parents fight or separate or divorce or witnessing domestic violence in one's childhood might be responsible for this phobia. Often, rejection in romantic love was so traumatic for the person, that they are not able to risk falling in love again. The heartache is just too painful.

~ Fear of commitment due to a few failed relationships, constant negative thoughts, anxiety and panic disorders are also linked to this phobia. People who are overly anxious or high strung might be more prone to it.

~ In many cultures and religions, having love relationships are seen as sin. The beliefs can be so serious that people are punished brutally if such norms are broken. This can create such extreme fear and anxiety in a person that it is impossible for them to fall in love.

~ Depression can be a major factor making it impossible for someone to focus on having a relationship and it can affect one's self-esteem negatively. If a person has been depressed, they are more vulnerable and likely to isolate themselves from people and avoid any loving relationships.

Common symptoms occurring in philophobia are:

~ extreme anxiety and fear of falling in love or getting into a relationship;
~ suppressing inner feelings as much as possible;
~ complete avoidance of places where couples are found such as parks and movie theaters;
~ avoiding marriage and others' wedding ceremonies as well;
~ isolation from the external world due to the fear of falling in love; and

~ Physical signs such as shaking, racing heartbeat, trouble breathing, sweating, numbness, nausea, and even fainting when confronted with anything associated with love and romance. (16)

Some of the treatments for philophobia include but are not limited to Cognitive Behavioral Therapy. CBT is the most common treatment for philophobia. CBT helps the person explore their underlying thoughts on what can happen if they do fall in love. The talk therapy helps the sufferer look at the cause of their anxiety and teaches them how to overcome it.

Exposure Therapy is another promising treatment. The therapist helps the individual role play by putting the client in situations replicating events that would represent interactions of being on a date and in romantic situations.

In the most extreme situations, medications may be recommended along with talk therapy.

Hypnosis is a viable tool in helping you to overcome the fear of falling in love. Through hypnosis you can get to the root cause that triggered your reaction to falling in love. Oftentimes, one may think they know the root cause, but through hypnosis they may discover that the root cause is another event altogether.

Please do not let fear of love destroy your chance of finding love and knowing the joy that comes with being in love, loving another person, and being loved by that person.

How can you deal with fear and prevent it from destroying your chance at finding a loving and supportive partner?

1. Label the underlying fear. It is a fear of falling in love, fear of rejection, fear of loss, fear of change, or lack of control. Possibly it is an expectation of failure being overwhelmed, a feeling of helplessness and of being ignored.
2. Share these concerns with your potential partner. Own your anxiety instead of blaming the other person.

3. Listen to the other person's fears. Often, they have the same apprehensions that you have, but are in better control of their emotions. By having this conversation, you may find that you are not alone and that you will be supported in the exploration of discovering where this relationship will take you.

4. Recognize that your potential partner's fears can also trigger your anxiety. Open and honest discussion about your concerns can help build a bond between the two of you.

5. Focus on the trepidation that you are feeling. Do not get sidetracked by specific details.

6. Keep the distress in check. Keep the discussion on track and do not linger in the discussion. Keep it within a reasonable time frame.

Metaphysical science teachers tell us that love is found in the fourth chakra which is our heart chakra. Our heart chakra is located in the center of our body. It is our "central command center" so to speak. Interesting isn't it that the chakra connecting the physical body to the spiritual body is located in the center of the chest. We think that our conscious mind is in control, but, in reality, it only thinks it is. The heart knows everything, the mind knows nothing when it comes to emotions. It is from our heart that spiritual lessons emerge and lessons are taught about love and compassion. It is from our heart that the most powerful universal energy emits the power of love.

This is the Divine energy that pours out endless nurturing of love from the life-force of Creator God. From this chakra comes the sacrament of Marriage. The first representation of marriage is the bond with one's internal union of self and soul. We cannot bond with another person successfully if we have not bonded with our own self. We have to know who we are and we have to love ourselves before we can love someone else.

The challenge we face with our heart chakra is our feelings about our internal world. Our emotional response to our thoughts, ideas, attitudes, and inspirations is vital as we give attention to our emotional needs. Until we are able to have a healthy connection with our internal self and our soul, we cannot form a healthy relationship with others. It is essential that we have this level of commitment to ourselves, if we want to have a deep healthy relationship with others.

To make that connection with our internal self can be difficult. We want to see the person who we project to the public. To see who we really are is hard. It's not necessarily hard because our internal self has a dark side. Our internal self may be filled with light, but we have been taught that if we acknowledge the good we have to offer is to be conceited and arrogant. We are taught if we love ourselves we are separating ourselves from God. Self-love is sinful and pious.

There are some primary fears that can prevent us from forming a loving relationship with another person. Fears of loneliness, commitment, the fear of not being able to protect our heart from possible betrayal, and the fear of emotional weakness can keep us from moving forward in finding a truly loving connection.

For some of us, falling in love is as easy as turning on a light switch. Love comes easily and often. People who are able to fall in love at the drop of a hat know the sting of rejection. They have learned that there is a risk in falling in love and they are willing to take it. They have learned to work through rejection a little faster than the rest of us.

The primary strengths we learn from the heart chakra are unconditional love, forgiveness, compassion, hope, trust, and the ability to heal not only ourselves, but others.

This Divine power found in the heart chakra is, in truth, the power center because *Love Is The Divine Power* living within us. Unconditional love is the purest form of love and is the wealth and abundance of the Divine which gives us the ability to be forgiven and it responds to our prayers. It is our spiritual nature to express compassion and forgiveness through love.

First John 4:18 (NIV) tells us that: There is no fear in love. But perfect love drives out fear, because fear has to do with punishment. The one who fears is not made perfect in love.

Jeremiah 29:11 reminds us: "For I know the plans I have for you," declares the LORD, "plans to prosper you and not to harm you, plans to give you hope and a future."

Father God wants us to experience not only His love, but the love of a romantic relationship. He wants us to have the companionship of a helpmate, a soulmate. There is no greater love than the love God has for us, but He offers us the love and support of a companion to walk through life with. Trust in Father's judgment and embrace the love of a life partner once you have found it. Do not let fear keep you in the gripping bondage of philophobia. Do not lose the opportunity of loving someone and being loved by them. The rewards of unconditional love are available to you. Do not suffer from the regret of love lost.

There has been more articles and books written on love than any other topic. Love has different meanings to different people. Love is nurturing, accepting, is patient, compassionate, and forgiving. Love heals the soul and the individual.

1 Corinthians 13:4–8 4 Love is patient, love is kind. It does not envy, it does not boast, it is not proud. 5 It does not dishonor others, it is not self-seeking, it is not easily angered, it keeps no record of wrongs. 6 Love does not delight in evil but rejoices with the truth. 7 It always protects, always trusts, always hopes, always perseveres. 8 Love never fails. But where there are prophecies, they will cease; where there are tongues, they will be stilled; where there is knowledge, it will pass away. (NIV)

We hear "time heals all wounds" but that is not necessarily true. However, love does heal all wounds. When it seems that our life is out of harmony and perfection, that is the time to invite the Angel of Love to oversee the repair to our emotional and spiritual wounds. The Angel of Love shows us unconditional love. Love without judgment, reservation, or question. It accepts us just as we are, no matter what.

Unconditional love is a hard concept for humans to comprehend and even harder to put into practice. Loving others unconditionally may not change the person being loved, but the true gift is that we are transformed. When we love unconditionally, we have created an atmosphere of making positive changes easier.

Because love is so powerful, we have to learn of love's intensity in stages. We first learn about love through our family, but at times this lesson is not easily learned because our family may not be able to express unconditional love to others. In most cases, love is an energy that is shared among the family members.

The second thing we learn about love is through our friends and other people we come in contact with as we grow into adulthood. We learn to love through bonds of friendship and learn how to express loyalty to include people outside of our family.

The third area we learn about love is through the appreciation of external experiences such as seeing a beautiful sunset with its glorious colors of red, pink, and tinges of orange. Seeing the miracle of the birth of a newborn life is one of the most joyful moments in life.

It is through this third lesson we learn about love by dating other people and making more intimate and emotional connections.

What happens, if as a child, we are wounded by those who are not able to show love to us? All of us have had to experience painful events in our lives when we were rejected in love. The shadow side of the emotions of fear of abandonment becomes jealousy and sexual abuse which becomes dysfunctional sexuality.

It is these types of situations that cause a false negative sense of self-esteem. These patterns can damage our emotional relationships with others, both personally and professionally. It affects our health negatively as well.

Healing is possible through forgiveness. It is a necessity to forgive before we are able to heal. Self-love is caring for ourselves enough so that we can forgive the people in our past who have hurt us. By releasing these wounds, we are enabled to move forward and participate with God in learning to act out of love and compassion instead of fear.

How do we heal the wounds from lost love? How do we move beyond the "needy" state into a healthy state of being? How can we bring power back into our life? How can we heal a broken heart? Is it really possible to pull yourself out of the "quicksand of grief" that is sucking you under and threatening your life, your very existence? There are steps that you can take to free yourself from the quicksand that is pulling you down deeper into disparity.

Healing is not easy, but it is not complicated either. Here are some steps you can take to heal:

1. Decide that you want to heal and commit yourself to the healing process. This will mean that you will have to reflect on what has happened and acknowledge the pain within you. You have to see your pain for what it is and give a name to it.

2. Identify the emotions that are associated with the pain. Have you given your power over to the pain? If you have given your personal power over to the pain, you will have to confront why you are afraid to heal yourself. Have you allowed the pain to be who you now are? Is the pain how you identify yourself? You are not the pain. It is not who you are. As you identify the pain, have someone you trust review it with you. This person

will be able to influence you in releasing the pain that has kept you in bondage.

3. Once you have verbalized your pain and see it for what it really is, notice how you use the pain to manipulate and control the people around you as well as yourself. Are you afraid that if you release the pain and allow yourself to heal you will lose your intimate connection of being the victim? If you let go of the pain, are you afraid to heal yourself because you will be required to leave that part of your life behind?

4. Identify why you are fearful of becoming healthy. It is hard to give up old patterns that no longer serve you. What do we put in that space once we release the pain? See the good that has come from your pain. Give thanks for the pain, in doing so, you are able to come to know that growth comes out of the pain. By showing gratitude for the painful experience you had in love, you are allowing yourself to grow as an individual and by recognizing the pain you are able to move out of the victim stage.

5. Consciously appreciate where you have been. Once you are able to do this, you are then ready to begin the healing process of forgiveness. Forgiveness is the conscious act that will liberate you from seeing yourself as a powerless victim. Forgiveness also means releasing the control that the perception of victimhood has over you. This liberation of forgiveness helps you to transition into a higher state of consciousness and allows you to establish a new beginning.

6. Think on love and appreciation and gratitude. When you invite this change into your life, your attitude will begin to change. Once this happens, you are free to enjoy unconditional love and know what true love is really like. You have allowed yourself to heal.

Our heart is the epicenter of our energy source, it is the essence of who we really are. Everyone will experience heartbreak at some point in life. Regardless of how broken your heart is, it is your choice on what you will do about healing it. Only you can liberate yourself. No one else can save you, no one else can heal you. The question remains the same: What will you do with the pain of lost love? Life will continuously present an opportunity for you to discover who you are and to love yourself. What will you do with that opportunity?

Too often people are frightened to learn who they really are and they convince themselves that if they learn the truth, they will be alone in life. We cannot attain a higher level of consciousness until we know who we are. We cannot know who we are until we learn to love ourselves. Once we learn to love ourselves, then we are able to break the chains that have held us captive and free ourselves to once again love others.

The Angel of Love profoundly works within us in the vibration of love and compassion. Our spirit flourishes as the Angel of Love nourishes our very being. The change has come from within us, helping us to offer love, compassion, and trust to others through God's care and love toward us. We have Creator's guidance showing us unconditional love to be used for the highest purpose, for the highest good for all. As we learn how to show unconditional love we are enabled to love more fully in many ways.

PRAYER

I cry out to the Angel of Love and my guardian angel to assist me in understanding the true concept of unconditional love. Guide me to help others understand unconditional love. The love given with no strings attached and with no expectations. Aid me as I release the selfish confines of immature love, the love that does not allow another to grow. Assist me as I take notice of my own heart, seeing the evolution by the expression of unconditional love.

As the Angel of Love stands next to me, gently directing me in the ways of unconditional love, I pray that others will see the light and love of the one and only Divine Love radiating outward from me.

Teach your children of your love and teach them that unconditional love is not an expression to manipulate them. Grant your children the understanding to trust unconditional love for what it is, unconditional. Remove the doubt humankind has with the phrase of "unconditional love."

Angel of Love, I ask that this distrust be released as mankind learns the true meaning of being loved unconditionally. Thank you for your example of unconditional love toward me.

Was Adam able to work past his fear of rejection in love? I do not know. The ending is yet to be written. Let's pray that he is able to embrace the love of a lifetime.

10

Why Should I Forgive You?
How Can I Forgive You?

"I might forgive him, but I'll never forget what he did."
Most of us have heard someone make this statement.
Some of us have even said it to ourselves. In either case, we are
not alone.

You have been deeply hurt. You did not deserve to be hurt.
Your agony runs so deep that you think you will never be able
to pull out the taproot. It has tunneled so deep that it causes a
festering wound. It seems this inflamed wound will never heal,
not even with the distance of time.

The distress reappears just when you think it is gone. There
seems to be nothing you can do to free yourself from this excruciating suffering. We have become cocooned within the pain
and are afraid to emerge.

Is there nothing that can be done to free ourselves from this
pain and suffering? Are we doomed to be forever the slaves of

our emotions? How can you end this recurring cycle of despair? Is there to be no reconciliation between the person who inflicted the suffering onto you and with you?

There is a way to stop the festering heartache of emotional distress. It is called forgiveness. Surely reconciliation can't be that hard or can it?

Christ taught us forgiveness through love. To forgive is one of the harder requirements of love. We have to deal with a storm of complex emotions. Forgiveness as a conscious, deliberate decision to release feelings of resentment or vengeance toward a person or group of people who have mistreated you, regardless of whether they actually deserve your forgiveness or not. Can we really forgive and put the emotional pain behind us? Can we forget? Can we move forward and away from the injustice done to us? How do we reconcile with those who have wounded us?

There are ten steps we can take to work through and to achieve our goals of forgiveness and reconciliation.

~ The first step in forgiveness is expressing your feelings. Torment is usually the dominant emotion we have. The deep down hurt felt by the betrayal rips us apart inside.

Express your grief. This can be done by writing down how you feel or you may want to talk about your sorrow with a trusted friend. You may want to imagine that you are in a safe environment and act out your struggle by imagining that the other person is present. Tell the individual how their actions hurt you. Be honest with yourself and the other person. This exercise in imagining your meeting with the person who hurt you is very beneficial. This imagined meeting will help you work through your feelings in a safe environment by letting you fully express your pain. You are better able to work out your emotions by identifying what your feelings truly are.

The most important aspect in this step is to be totally honest. It does not matter how hateful your feelings seem. Honesty with yourself is the only way to work through the betrayal you feel.

While working through your feelings seek God's help. Express your feelings to God and ask Him to help you work through these intrusive feelings that just do not want to seem to leave you alone.

Keep in mind that it takes time to work through these feelings of strife. You are not a failure if it takes days or weeks or months to deal with the pain.

~ The second step is decide to forgive and pray. Do you want to be healed or do you want to continue to suffer? Hate is a natural response to an unjustified act of betrayal against you. Instinctively we want revenge and to prove ourselves righteous. When we hate people who have wronged us, our hostility continues to live within us, to spiral out of control. Our loathing of the other person can divide our own soul, to bring us into conflict with ourselves. One part of our soul detests the person who hurt us, the other part of our soul wants to hold onto the love that we had for this individual. But we must remember, a divided house falls.

Animosity eventually must be healed. Holding on to resentment by nurturing and tending to it in an active hostility toward the other person will, in time, defeat you. If it is not healed it expands into a debilitating life crisis; it will destroy you if you hold on to it.

Forgiveness, like love, is a decision, not a matter of feeling. Making the decision to forgive will not change your feelings automatically. But what will happen is that you begin to notice that you are dwelling on the memory of the pain less and less. It begins to fade into the past where it belongs.

Admit to God that you do not feel like forgiving and that you feel hateful toward the other person. Admit that you need help in forgiving. You may have to pray about this for several days or weeks or months to overcome the malice you feel.

Remember, forgiveness is a process. It takes time, but if your prayers are sincere, Creator God will place the desire to forgive in your heart.

~ The third step is to confess and repent. Ask yourself: "Was there anything in my behavior that caused the other person to act in the manner they did? Do I harbor resentments and grudges toward the other person?" There are two sides to the story. Your side of the story, their side of events, and somewhere in the middle lies the truth. It is seldom one person's fault in any situation. Look deep within yourself and be honest about your part in the event. Yes, it will be painful to see the shadow side of your role you played in the incident.

As long as we focus on the other person's actions we do not make much progress. Often it helps to confess our own sins and let the other person worry about his sins.

Repentance is a gift. We need to pray for the grace to be truly sorry for our feelings of harm we have for the other person. Ask Source to help you have a more loving attitude toward this person. Each and every person who turns to God in genuine repentance and faith will be saved and blessed by placing their trust in Father to help them learn and grow from the experience.

~ In step four we let go of fear and anger. As a defense, we harden our hearts when we have been injured. We do not want to take the first step in reconciliation, because we fear rejection. Sometimes our basic reaction is anger instead of fear. When we neglect to deal with anger, we have little desire to reach out to the other person.

When dealing with a heart of stone, we have to ask God to soften our heart. Since we are often helpless in the effort to change our hearts, we learn to trust Father God to do the work for us.

We must let Spirit have the fear and anger. The wall we have built around our heart must come down. If we keep taking it back He cannot do his work.

~ Step five teaches us to gain a fair perspective. Forgiveness is like spiritual surgery. You must cut away the wrong that was done to you. Let go of the hurt. Let the wound heal from within moving outward, to be filled up with the love and light of Father God.

The more we think about the injustice inflected on us, the more we tend to exaggerate the size of the emotional wound. We become blind to our part in the conflict. By accommodating these feelings, we have locked ourselves into an eternity loop filled with emotional suffering.

By releasing the pain we gain new insight. We see that the person who caused us distress is weak, needy, and fallible. When we see this, we are able to forgive them and that gives us new feelings about the humanity of the individual involved. We also have renewed feelings about ourselves.

You may have to be content with the healing inside of you. You may forgive them, but you may not be able to reestablish the relationship. Still, when you forgive you are healed.

~ In step six we imagine a meeting. To reestablish the relationship, both of you must bring about an honest coming together.

Before meeting with the other person try praying for them. Then imagine meeting with the other person in a neutral space where you feel protected. Tell them of your desire to reestablish your relationship. A heartfelt attempt to reconnect with the individual is usually appreciated by your former comrade and companion.

The imagined conference may seem strange, but there is a great benefit in this acting out of the meeting. In acting out the imagined appointment in your mind, you will be working through the details that you would like to see as the result of your encounter with your friend. One will have more confidence during the actual meeting because needed steps to reach the goal have been identified before hand.

~ Step seven finds us actually meeting with the other person. Hold out your hand to the other person in an attempt to resolve this conflict. In this reconciliation you both must bring truthfulness and sincerity to the table for discussion.

Without truthfulness, this coming together will not have much meaning. Nicely timed and sincerely meant, the humble and graceful apology is a gesture that helps us better deal with each other and to learn to appreciate each other's unique qualities.

Should apologies be accepted in place of repentance? Should we forgive someone who does not repent? Yes, we must free ourselves of the conflict for our own sake. We need to realize that others have to be responsible for themselves and their own emotions.

Leave the revenge to Creator God. Your forgiveness is just as real, you have healed yourself.

~ Step eight brings us to thanksgiving. Give thanks to Him for helping you work through the conflict. Giving thanks helps us to remember that all good things come from God our Father. By giving thanks, we stimulate a healing environment. Gratitude is not only a feeling of thankfulness and appreciation; but also an act that will bring us closer to ALL-THAT-THERE-IS and trusting Him to resolve the situation with a perfect outcome for both parties involved.

~ In step nine we find a deepening in forgiveness and reconciliation. The initial act of forgiveness and reconciliation will need to be supported by other acts of love. Ask I AM to protect the reunion you have reestablished with your friend. By taking the action to rectify the situation we find that the restoration of friendly relations has helped us to grow spiritually.

~ Step ten shows us how impossible forgetting may be. To "forgive and forget" may not exclude emotions of anger after the forgiving. You are not a failure if after you forgive you still feel angry at times. In time, you will, however, notice that the memory and anger felt during the initial conflict have become more distant in your remembrance of the circumstance.

When you remember the hurt, you can be angry without hatred. Anger without hate is a sign that your forgiveness is real. Your anger can prevent the same wrong from happening again. The frustration you felt during the conflict can act as a warning sign in the future to help prevent the same kind of conflict from reoccurring.

The only way you can heal the pain is to overlook the act of the person who hurt you. Forgiving stops the remembering of the betrayal and pain. When you cut the pestilence from your spirit, fill the space with God's light and peace of mind and you will find that a true healing has taken place.

Given time and the love of Universal Spirit we cannot only pardon this action, but in a spiritual sense forget. Release of the pain is possible.

Forgiveness is the key to happiness, the key to peace of mind. It is not enough to excuse someone for having done something you disagree with and who has hurt you, but you must forgive them as well. You have to forgive yourself for your misconception of that person, for judging that person and not seeing them as a loving human being. Once we see the other person as a child of God, then we can release the guilt.

Jesus seems to imply that unwillingness to pardon transgression is the cause of many losing their souls. In Matthew 18:21–35 NIV, Peter asked Jesus how often must we forgive, and Jesus answers "seventy times seven." Then the disciples cried out, "Lord, increase our faith. If we have to be that forgiving, we need more Faith." Then, to help their faith, Jesus speaks of the Unlimited Power of Faith, and then by the parable of the obedient servant shows them that Humility is the groundwork of Faith.

Do you want to be completely and throughly healed? Do you want to be whole? Health is a matter of wholeness. Health is more than being physically fit. It is being emotionally, mentally, and spiritually fit as well.

Have you become an invalid? As invalids we say, "I can't." Mentally we become a victim and refuse to acknowledge our participation in our invalid state.

Do you feel that you are not able or are you unwilling to receive the love from someone else, from God? Do you want to be healed?

Jesus will not deal with invalids as though we are a victim. He will teach us to take responsibility for our lives and participate in our own healing. He expects us to do our part by taking action to move forward and become whole again.

Yahweh, The Lord God who sees and knows us in our incapacitated state reaches out to us. He invites us, with deep compassionate love and concern, to release our powerful desires, to rise up with the reparative power of wholeness, and to participate in our recovery. He then invites us to go beyond our own restorative state, by reaching out to others and helping them in their own personal attempts at restoration.

How can we help someone else in their battle to heal when we are struggling in prayer about our own needs? Our own prayer life takes such an effort at times that it takes all our energy just to utter a short prayer. Prayer can be a source of frustration when we are having difficulty focusing on what we want to say to God. Our mind wanders, we repeat ourselves, we question whether or not the Lord even hears our prayers. Praying is hard during these moments and at times it seems mystical. Is there a formula for praying? Can we be successful when we pray?

Before we begin to pray, we need to take a few moments of solitude so we can become focused and detach from the distractions of the day. We need to quieten our mind and transition into the process of prayer. We need to make sure that we are in the right frame of mind before we start to pray. Listening to soft music or religious music can assist us with the transition. Meditation can help focus the mind and prepare the mind and heart for communication with God.

Rabbi Ariel Bar Tzadok tells us in his writing on The Secrets of Successful Prayers: That prayer "stands in the high places of the universe." Prayer is one of the most important and powerful tools known to man. (11)

When we stand in the high places of universal love, we stand in the presences of a loving, compassionate, and forgiving God. He has lifted us up to a higher vibrational level and invited us to sit at His table to have communion with Him.

Intercession should be focused on meaningful thought, not trivial wishes such as "I want to win the billion dollar lottery."

Many religions teach that there is a certain element of prayer preparation and that there are steps one must take before we can talk with God. There are many steps that we must take before we can even think about talking with our Creator, according to many theologians.

What did Jesus teach us about prayer? Jesus taught us the most effective prayer is the 'Lord's Prayer'. He taught us to go into the closet to pray. The closet has different meanings in different religions, but the meaning is two-fold. First, to 'go into the closet' is to commune with the Lord without drawing attention to oneself. Do not make a big production in praying even when you are called on to pray for a group of people. The second meaning of 'go into the closet' is that of entering the quiet space of one's mind and connecting your mind with the mind-set of I AM THAT I AM, I WILL BE WHO I WILL BE.

In his book, *I Will Lift Up Mine Eyes*, Glenn Clark tells the story about the hind, also known as the mountain deer. This animal travels on steep mountain ridges where one misstep would result in the hind falling to its death. The hind's feet track true. The back feet track true to the front feet. In other words, the back feet will tract in the exact spot where the front feet tracked. In his analogy of the hind's feet tracking true, Mr. Clark talks about our conscious mind and subconscious mind tracking true one to the another. If we align our conscious mind with our subconscious mind, then we are able to accomplish anything that is our heart's truest desire. Glenn Clark uses the Lord's Prayer to walk us through thoughtful conversation with Spirit and aligning our conscious and subconscious minds one to the other.

Glenn Clark gives us tools to help us pinpoint what steps we need to take to determine what our heart's truest desires are and how to take steps to move toward this goal.

The first tool he gives us are the 'Seven Whatsoever Checks in the Bank of God'. These whatsoever checks teach us to ask for:

1. Divine Spirit to enter us and fill us completely.
2. To pray for Thy kingdom to come, in earth as it is in heaven.
3. Pray for my will to become completely and utterly His will.
4. To pray for my actual needs to be met by the right supply, in the right way, and at the right time.
5. He tells us to ask for the right people to come into our life, at the right time and in the right way.
6. We should pray for the right ideas to come to us in perfect sequence and in perfect order, in the right time, and in the right way.
7. Lastly, he tells us to pray for our deepest soul's desire to be filled in the right time and in the right way.

Jesus teaches us that the "Kingdom of God is within us" which is referring to a state of consciousness. This state of consciousness is a creative force that is not stagnant, it grows and expands with divine light from the soul within us outward into the universe. The Kingdom of Heaven is a state of peace and permanent harmony. Being in the Kingdom of Heaven starts out so infinitesimally small that we may not realize we have even planted the seed. Soon, this seed grows, spreading its vines, reaching ever upward to higher heights of enlightenment advancing throughout us to the point that it has filled us completely with the consciousness of divine love.

Next Glenn Clark talks about these three "Anything checks":

~ Grant to me the power to love everybody and everything.
~ Grant to me the capacity to see everything as intensely and ecstatically beautiful.
~ Grant to me the ability to see infinite value and importance in everything that God has made.

How do we align ourselves with God? To align ourselves with I AM, we have to make our will His will. How do we make our will His will? We must be willing to form a partnership with Him. We do this by meeting Lord God halfway. When we asked for the right people to come into our life at the right time, and in the right way, we have to be open to receiving these people into our life. Sometimes, when the right person comes into our life, we may not recognize that this person is, indeed, who we have been praying for, they may seem to be someone we would not have interacted with during our daily activities.

To make our will Creator's will requires that we surrender ourselves to Source and let Him take the lead. We need to make sure that our intention is right and God will take care of the result. This means that whoever or whatever I AM decides is the best result for us, we have to be open to receiving that blessing.

When we say, "I will to will the will of God" we have to realize that there are three wills in the sentence. The first will is the mankind will, the third will is the Creator's will, and the second will is the will-in-action. The first and third wills unite in perfect harmony and bring forth the second will of manifesting itself into action.

When our conscious mind and subconscious mind align they become as hind's feet. Anything is now possible. Think about what it is that you want in your life, are you in need of a different job, one that will offer you the opportunity to be creative, to earn a higher salary? If you have been diligent and learned the skills for this job, then you need to take the following steps to manifest your heart's truest desires:

1. Imagine in your mind seeing your heart's desire. Hold onto this image as you visualize this desire. If it is a different job, envision the job that you want, see it clearly within your mind's eye. Holding onto the image of seeing yourself in this position that you want will move you forward toward acquiring this goal.

2. Notice the good feeling that you have when you are thinking about this job. Really feel the excitement, the joy, and the pleasure that this position brings into your heart. Letting these good feelings anchor and take hold in your subconscious mind is the beginning of having "hind's feet."

3. Next, release your heart's truest desire into the hands of Father. Let our Creator help you manifest this true desire and bring it to fruition. (12)

Keep in mind that there is no limitation to the abundance that the universe has to offer to us. Resources are not limited as we have been taught. Our Provider has no limits on resources and He will not limit our prosperity that He desires to bring into our life.

Metaphysical law teaches us that the universe holds an unlimited supply of abundance ready for our receiving. This unlimited supply of good is for everyone. Each one of us can enjoy the abundance of prosperity of health and love.

Genuine prosperity is living in harmony with divine love. When we are living in divine love, we find that we have set things right in the spiritual plane and, in doing so, we have aligned things correctly on the material plane.

Divine love dismisses all fears. For out of fear rises poverty, illness, worries, and negative thoughts. Consciously eliminate negative thoughts concerning any form of "lack." Deny the "lack" of attitude and replace it with affirmation of abundance. Remember, your thoughts are prayers. Knowing that words have great power and that when we think or speak works of poverty, this is what we are creating in our own reality. Our words and thoughts set universal forces into motion, so, in order to have the best outcomes in our life make sure your words and thoughts are of a positive nature. What we think and believe is what we will see manifest in our lives.

The Angel of Abundance is ready to assist us to position ourselves to bring our consciousness into sequence with the mind-set of Divine Source. Once we are aligned with Source, we are able to establish a link of energy to connect us with the conscious field of universal abundance. Properly attuned with Creator by using affirmations and prayer in constructive ways, we declare what we seek has already manifested. Through this prayer we have set in motion the energetic forces that enable us to manifest our affirmation. What we desire, we think, we believe, and then we see it manifested into our life. To claim these gifts from Father, we use our affirmations to expand our horizons beyond all limitations. Abundance is ours when we keep our thoughts centered on God.

PRAYER

Angel of Abundance and my guardian angel, please guide me as I become aware of my connection to All-That-There-Is. I request that this connection will never be broken. I pray that I will never be separated from the limitless perfection of abundance and infinite love. Help me to realize that true abundance is in knowing God and being known by Him. Help me to remember abundance is more than financial wealth. Abundance is foremost the love and compassion of Spirit Most High.

How do we develop powerful prayers? Can we pray powerful prayers? What happens when we pray powerful prayers?

11

Powerful Prayers

"Seek ye first the kingdom of God and His rightness, and all these things shall be added unto you.

"The kingdom of God is within you," Jesus said.

How does one enter into the kingdom of God? Why would we want to enter into the kingdom of God? Is there really a kingdom of God?

We enter into the dominion of God in a state of consciousness. Individually each of us enters into His holy house through prayer. How can one personally enter the realm of God through prayer? Why does it seem that prayer works for some and not others?

Praying is not mystical, nor is it something that is hard to do. You and I do not have to talk in formal language when we communicate with Source. Remember, prayer is communication between you and your Creator, an intimate interaction, using your own words. Communication is a learned art. It takes time to develop these skills. Patience and practice are needed, but we do learn the art of effective conversation.

Jesus talked about prayer on many occasions. He taught us to pray when he said the Lord's Prayer. Jesus also showed us how to communion with Father.

So, why is it that there is such difficulty putting into practice what Jesus taught? Maybe part of the problem is our desire for someone else to tell us what to say or ask for, or we just want them to do the praying for us. We become lazy, it is easier to read a prayer than to speak from the inner recesses of our soul. Perhaps part of the problem is we live in a hurry-up world and God does not hurry. Or, maybe, part of the problem is we feel differently in our hearts. At times it seems hopeless to pray. It is just too hard!

Jesus spoke of going into the closet to pray. This should be our first step, find a quiet place. Clear the mind of the worries and problems of the day. I know at times it is almost impossible to free our mind of the constant chatter that seems to just go on and on. How do we get into a prayerful mood? Reading from the Bible or your religion's holy book can help you as you transfer your thoughts from the day's worries and concerns to thoughts of God the Supreme Being. Listening to religious or mediative music can help us unwind from the tensions of the day. It can help to uplift our spirits by bringing us to a higher vibrational level, a higher level closer to God. Looking upward into the heavens at the stars can bring us into the presence of Creator God as we see the wondrous majesty of His mastery in the wisdom of the universe.

As we slip into a prayerful state of mind, our soul is then ready to move into the second step.

Jesus taught us to forgive those who have hurt us. This is very important. If you are angry or hate just one person, then you, yourself are separated from God Himself by that much. If you have not forgiven those who have wounded your soul, how can Father forgive you? When we are angry with an individual, we need to pray for that person. We need to give praise for this situation because it is showing us a side of ourselves that we do not want to see or acknowledge. It has opened us up to seeing the possibilities of our shadow side. One does not want to admit to ourselves that we too could do such a thing to hurt someone else. By giving praise and showing gratitude, we also realize that we are just as guilty as the person who inflicted pain on us. We are humbled in the acknowledgment of our own imperfection.

Hatefulness is the mightiest hindrance in our connecting with Spirit; anger toward a single individual can block every door to Father God. Fear is perhaps the greatest tension. Fear is a greater separative force from our King of Kings than many sins. Self-pity or self-conceit is also a big roadblock between us and a loving Father.

The power of blood is the power of love. Blood can bring recovery to the wounds of the body. Love has the power to heal the wounds of the personality, the soul, and the heart. Blood has the power to heal broken-down tissues and bring about restoration. Let the blood and love of Jesus Christ cleanse and heal your wounds physically, mentally, emotionally, and spiritually.

Once your own wounds have been healed and your separation from Yahweh has been dealt with, we are then ready to move on to the next step. Seek His guidance. How do we seek Our Lord's guidance?

Guidance comes through:

1. God's own word,
2. Outer circumstances (doors are opened or closed to us),
3. Your own best reasonable thinking,
4. The counsel of other like-minded people, and
5. The inner voice of your heart.

Ask The Source of Life to show you the divine inner plan for your own life. Ask Him to reveal to you the perfect sequence and order in such a way as to bring the greatest good to the greatest number of those involved in any circumstance.

Are your conscious desires integrated with your subconscious desires? Are the things you are desiring and praying for true to your own nature? Every mature desire that is whole, sincere, complete, and above all, which acknowledges its relationship to our Creator God, is always a good desire.

If you want to know His plan for you, ask Him. God is always ready to give a bountiful supply of wisdom to all who ask. But when one asks Him, be sure that you really expect Him to answer your request. If you have a doubtful mind, every decision made will be uncertain. If we do not ask with faith, do not expect God to give you any solid answers.

Then, wait on the Lord to take you forward. It is not God's way to give more light on the future than we need for action in the present, or to guide us more than one step at a time. When you are in doubt, do nothing. When action is needed, the answer will come. Remember, trouble is not necessarily a sign that you are off track. I AM sometimes allows us to be in the midst of trouble so that we may learn skills and gain knowledge from our mistakes. He allows us to have new experiences so we can grow in understanding on the ways of life.

The inward voice of the Spirit does not decide and dictate everything for us. Creator God gave us a brain and some brawn to work through problems. He also gave us free will to decide whether or not we want to follow Him.

God uses our sins and mistakes to let us learn, grow in knowledge, and mature. He does not shield us from assaults by the world, nor does he protect us from troubles created by our own temperament; by exposing us to our own sense of inadequacy, we learn to seek His wisdom. Troubles ensure that we will learn to depend on Him.

Then give praise. People who give praise to Father for all they have and for the beauty surrounding them are happier and see results from the seeds that they planted manifest sooner in their lives. Praise does not wait for results. It speaks out with joy and enthusiasm. Give God credit for all that you have, all that you are able to do, all that you are, and all that you hope to be. Then, again when your prayer is answered, your gratitude and praise should be in measure to the greatness of the power of which you have witnessed.

However, there is one thing about which you must be very careful, and that is: Do not interfere with His action by your worry and anxiety concerning the outcome. Worry is a prayer for something that you do not want to be manifested into your life in the future. To answer your request, He requires your absolute trust. Only through the avenue of a peaceful mind can God do His work.

For many of us, guidance is a fact, but at times we are not sure of it. Our concern is we may miss the guidance Creator God provides through some fault of our own. We become anxious because we are not certain of our receptiveness or ability to recognize the guidance All-That-There-Is has offered.

Our basic mistake is in thinking of guidance, as the strong inward prompting by the Holy Spirit, apart from the written Word. While intuition, the understanding of divine guidance is important, it is also important to know and discern the Word of God as well. Comprehension of the written word gives us insight into the nature of Father God. An insight that allows us to have an intimate relationship with our Creator God. A recognition of being known by God and knowing God, to draw us closer into His inner circle of love.

The problems of unanswered prayer:

1. We do not ask for the right things. We often pray with wrong motives. If these requests were answered it would not be for our highest good.

2. We ask for things we should be taking care of ourselves. We would not do the work our coworkers should be doing. God will not do our work either.

3. We are not ready for God's answer. We have not taken care of old business, so the time is not right. We have to release what no longer services us before we can move forward.

When our prayers seem to go unanswered, we need to examine our heart and our prayer. When we see that our intention is right, I AM THAT I AM, I WILL BE WHO I WILL BE, will look after the result.

Jesus asked, "How can I describe the kingdom of God? What story shall I use to illustrate it? It is like a tiny mustard seed! Though this is one of the smallest of seeds, yet it grows to become one of the largest plants, with long branches where birds can build their nests and be sheltered." (Mark 4:30–32 NIV)

Remember, we are dealing with the planting of prayers. The smaller and the more invisible your prayer effort, the greater the outflow of power. The more invisible your request, the more powerful it will become.

There are many ways to pray but two of the most common ways of praying is the John the Baptist way and the other is the way Jesus prayed.

John the Baptist had an extremely forceful way of praying. With John's prayer method you concentrate your thoughts upon your prayer subject and by tremendous strength and effort of thought you force the trouble to leave. John's method requires an immense amount of work and when you are through, you are exhausted. One who uses the method of John the Baptist's way of praying must be strong mentally, emotionally, and physically. Also, one will have to be knowledgeable in the laws of telepathy and mental therapeutics. This is exactly the type of prayer John used: Subliminal telepathy.

For centuries this form of communication has been proven. It is a very real and effective method which often produces results. But, it does have its limitations.

First, it requires an immense amount of work. Second, you are working in the "no man's land" of the psychic where bad thoughts can deflect the pure purpose of your prayer. Third, the results are not always lasting. The only way they are lasting is if you believe strongly in God or in the power of love or at least in the existence of a "friendly universe." John was the voice crying out in the wilderness. His energy force within him had the power behind it that could move a mountain. Very few of us today have that kind of powerful inner strength.

The method of Jesus sees only the Father and His Kingdom. With God, all troubles vanish. Jesus made this clear when he said, "Seek ye first the Kingdom of God. . . ." Jesus's method entails no work because our Father does all the work. This accounts for the fact that Jesus was regenerated after prayer. While Jesus's method does not require work in the way of doing things, it does require work in the way of being something.

Jesus described the difference between his method and that of John the Baptist in the first chapter of the Gospel of John. Nathanael was surprised that Jesus could read his thoughts and exclaimed, "Rabbi, Thou art the son of God; Thou art the king of Israel." Jesus replies that if Nathanael thinks it is wonderful that He can use the John the Baptist method of insight and read Nathanael's thoughts, he does not begin to know the wonders that he is going to see. Nathanael will be lifted into a heavenly insight where he "shall see heaven open, and the angels ascending and descending upon the Son of Man." Jesus is called the Word. The Word is with God. The Word is God.

Jesus's most revealing explanation came when he said, "I am the vine, ye are the branches: he that abideth in Me, and I in him, the same bringeth forth much fruit, for without Me ye can do nothing . . . If ye abide in Me and my words abide in you, ye shall ask what ye will, and it shall be done unto you . . . Herein is My Father glorified, that ye bear much fruit." (John 15:5)

We are one with Jesus and God and through this union is assurance of answered prayer.

Seeing the difference between the two methods of prayer, we would be wise to turn from the exhausting method that John the Baptist showed us and take up Jesus's method.

We enter into the kingdom of God in a state of consciousness. And when we enter into the kingdom of God, we enter into a powerful life through prayer.

In the book, *Sermon on the Mount: The Key To Success In Life* by Emmet Fox, we learn that Jesus did not teach theology. Jesus's teachings were of spiritual and metaphysical bases. Jesus taught us that focus is to be on the inner spiritual development of our connection with I AM THAT I AM and not on the outer observances of the world. In fact, the outer is just a manifestation of the inner. What we think, so it is. Remember, what you continue to think about to dwell on is what you will bring forth into your life.

Our thoughts that occupy our mind, our Secret Place, as Jesus referred to it, is molding our destiny for good or bad; the truth being said, is that everything we experience in life is the outer expression of our inner thoughts. Every thought we think is a prayer. Pay attention to your thoughts. Manifest only those thoughts which are of the highest good for all into reality. Wars are manifestations of thoughts, just as healing and love are manifestations of blessings. Guard your thoughts closely. Always be aware of where your thoughts are dwelling, what you are focused on, because the longer you reside in this thought pattern, the sooner you will see it transform into a reality of your life.

Religion teaches us that we are separated from God and that we are unworthy, unclean, sinful, and undeserving. We are taught that we fall short of God our Father's grace and love; that without Jesus we would never be worthy of His love or attention.

We are taught that even with Jesus in our life, we still are not worthy of God's love.

How can this be true if God our Creator made us in His image? Is God unworthy, unclean, sinful, and undeserving? He is the word of Love, He is Love, and He made us from Love. If we are created in Spirit's image and He is the word of Love, then how can we be anything other than an extension of His Love? We are like the innocent newborn, who is trusting the parents to take care of him and mold him to be the best person he can become. We, too, trust Our Father to take care of us and mold us into His image of what He knows we can become. Our Creator takes great pleasure in our spiritual growth, just as a parent takes pleasure in the development of their child.

Our consciousness is the one and only reality. It is the first and only foundation of the miracle of life. We attract into our reality health, wealth, wisdom, joy, and happiness. Like a magnet our subconscious mind will draw to us that which we dwell on in our thoughts. The subconscious mind, in its child-like acceptance, will absorb what the conscious mind directs it to. It does not matter if the thought is rational or not. Your concept of yourself and what you accept and consent to within your mind is your reality. Your reactions reveal where you are in your psychological maturity and determines how you live your life in the secular world.

By the renewing of your mind you are transformed. This is done by assuming the feeling of your desire. You can become the person you want to be by assuming that you already are that individual. If you are persistent with this assumption, then the reality of who you see yourself as will soon manifest into reality. Your attitude should be one in which having expressed this desire to a higher state of consciousness, the subconscious mind, you alone have accepted this act of incarnating this new and greater personification of who you now are.

Prayers are not successful unless there is a harmonious connection between the conscious and subconscious mind. This is done through having faith and using imagination. The idea that you desire and hope to bring forth into your life will not transpire into existence until you have imagined that you have already achieved that idea. Imagination and faith are the only tools needed to create positive outcomes.

To establish the rapport between the conscious and subconscious minds, focus your attention on the desired outcome. Imagine seeing the outcome fixed in your life. Next, feel the joy in witnessing this event unfold in your life and as having already been completed. Give thanks for this wonderful result. Remember, it is not what you want to happen that you will attract, but what you believe to be true. Jesus told us that, "whatsoever you desire, when you pray, believe that you received them, and you shall have them."

The subconscious mind is the universal lightning rod which we use to modify our thoughts and feelings. Self-confidence and the unmoved belief in the truth of our mental conviction are all that is needed to produce the expected results.

Successful prayer commands a clear defined objective of what you want before asking for it. You have to know what you want before you can feel that you have it. Prayer is the feeling of the dream becoming reality. To change your reality, first change your conception of what reality is. We are told that heaven is within us and we cannot receive anything unless it is given to us from heaven. Heaven is our subconscious mind. The habit of "talking to ourselves" is actually the most fruitful form of prayer when our thoughts are on those things which are of goodness for all involved.

Your attitude determines everything. If you do not believe in that idea and experience the feeling of having your desire by affirming that it is so, you will not have your heart's desire. Believing in the desire, having the attitude of its existence is necessary to achieve your goal. By imagining that you already experience what you desire, assuming the feeling that comes with owning this longing, then you will see the fulfillment of this burning dream come out of your consciousness.

To reach this higher level of being, one must assume a higher level of self-concept. By assuming the feeling of this wished desire as already being fulfilled makes the future today's reality.

Imagination is the beginning of all creation. Since your life is determined by the acceptance of your beliefs, then you have to recognize that you are either a slave to your presumptions or the master of your thoughts. To master your control over the conscious mind, form an image in the mind's eye and picture what it is that you desire in the person you want to become. Then feel yourself in that situation as though you are in those surroundings. By clearly imagining these circumstances you have changed your reality. Controlled imagination and firm attention that is repeatedly focused on the heart's desire are the secrets for success. You must deliberately focus all attention on the feeling of your desired wish until your mind is filled with this idea only. When we become still and know that what we desire is true, then it is firmly planted within us and we will not have to search for it.

Accept this wish as already being fulfilled. Once completely absorbed in this emotional state of knowing, you are at that moment transformed into the state of fulfillment. When you are intensely emotional about the dream of your heart's blessing, it is then that you will experience it in your world of reality. It is during these periods of complete absorption, of controlled concentration, that the seed is planted in the fertile soil of your mind that you will harvest the grains of life.

The Lord of All will not respond to your wish until you have taken responsibility of doing your part and assumed the feelings of already being who you want to be.

By taking the path of least resistance, you will use the minimum of energy and take the shortest possible amount of time in your journey from thought of the wish to be fulfilled into the reality of it being completed.

The future becomes present time when you imagine that what you want you have. Be still, know that you are now who you want to be. Perpetual construction of the future states that without the consciousness of already being who you intend to be is the fallacy and phantom of humankind.

The Angel of Prayer has one of the most important functions in connecting us to I AM so that we are communing with him. Archangels Sandalphon, Gabriel, and Raphael are instrumental in overseeing that prayers are delivered to God. These archangels have legions of angels helping to advance our prayers from one level to the next.

When we ask the Angel of Prayer to assist us, we are instantaneously connected to the angel who is most appropriate to help with our needs. Prayer enables us to make appropriate changes in our life. We are able to draw on Father's spiritual strength, courage, and inspiration through prayer. In this communing with God, our spirit is nourished and we are able to persevere in overcoming obstacles in our path.

When we pray, a conduit of spiritual energy is opened. This energy flows between us and the Divine Mind of Creation by restoring, strengthening, and revitalizing us. This love radiates out from us and becomes a beacon of light to draw others into the inner circle of Divine love. Prayer teaches us many things. Through prayer, we open our mind to the consciousness of the Divine to lift us to higher levels of knowledge. Our energy field is changed as the knowledge of God's love and power becomes known to us.

All prayers are answered. We may not like the answer or we may not understand the answer, but our prayer is answered. The possible answers are: Yes, or it is answered in another way, or no.

What does, "in another way" mean? When it seems that our prayer is not being answered, we need to look in another direction. Another way reminds one that there are other possibilities that our desired prayer will be answered. Our prayer is always answered to the highest good for us and all of those involved.

The answer "not yet" can be frustrating for us. Waiting for the right time can be difficult. What we need to realize is that there could be something blocking the way and it has to be resolved first. It could mean that we have not completed the preparation work that we were supposed to do. We have to do our own work. If one's prayer involves praying for others, you have to remember that the other person may not be open to receiving the healing that we have been praying for on their behalf.

Prayer should never be used to manipulate a situation or other people. It should never be uttered to harm someone else. Prayer should be spoken in love, compassion, and in the highest good for all involved.

The one and only purpose of prayer is to know God. God is the living word of Love. Once we are taken into His circle of love, we begin to know the Lord of Love and His Truth.

PRAYER

Angels of Prayer and my guardian angel, please hear my prayer and carry it to the heavenly seat of God Our Father for consideration. I open myself up to the answer that is in the highest interest for myself and others. I pay attention to the loving energy from God for the answer. I pray for the wisdom to recognize the completed answer that is being presented to me. I open my arms and my heart to receive the blessings Creator God wishes to bestow on me.

12

Called to the Knowledge of God

What is the biggest lie that humankind has been told? We have been told that we are separated from God. There has been a veil of separation placed between us and our Creator for centuries. The myth that we are not One with Lord God is an illusion. In reality, the one becomes the whole. There is no separation from God and as His children we are not separated from our Father. We are One, With All That There Is. The lie of separation is all a sham that we have been living with for centuries. This gully has kept us on the other side of the valley of love. It is preventing us from being able to see the love and light radiating across the valley of peaceful joy toward us.

When Moses came into the presence of the Flaming Bush, Moses asked God by what name shall I tell the people you are called. God proclaimed His name to be I AM THAT I AM. The expanded version of I AM is, I AM THAT I AM, I WILL BE WHO I WILL BE. Creator did not just tell us His name, but, made a declaration of who He is. Think about this name for a moment. Really think about it. When I AM revealed His name to us He gave insight into who He really is. We say that God is never changing, that He is today what He was in the beginning of time. But, is this true? Read His name again, *really read* and think about it. I AM THAT I AM, I WILL BE WHO I WILL BE. God's name implies that He is not stagnant. The second part of I AM's name tells us that He does grow and expand. We grow and expand with each new experience just as God expands with the changes in this world and the Universe. "I AM" is the Activity of "That Life." "I AM" is the full activity of God. Our Universe grows and expands and changes. New life comes into being as the Universe expands, creating lifeforms that had not been in existence before. (9)

According to Godfré Ray King, who channeled St. Germain in the early 1930s, we do not realize the full impact of the words I AM. If we did we would use these words with more thought of intention. It is hard for us to grasp the true meaning of these words. "I AM" is the Full Activity of God. "I AM" are the two most powerful words that we can ever speak.

When we say, "I AM not," we have stopped the flow of energy between us and God. Every time you say, "I AM not" or "I cannot," you have not only slowed or stopped the energy flow between you and Source, you set into motion an intention that you most likely did not intend. We have now established an outcome that we did not expect. We literally "will not" be able to or we literally "cannot" move forward in life. When you make a declaration of "I AM not," you have moved into a direction that will stagnate your abilities to manifest the goodness into your life that God intended you to have. On the flip side of this coin, we have to take care in using the words I AM. When we say, "I AM sick," then we have catapulted ourselves into illness. If we continue to say, "I AM poor," then this is what we will be. We are what we say. What we think is what we are. I cannot say this to you enough!

Mr. King tells us, "STOP! I say to you, giving power to the outer conditions, persons, places, or things, and in the Name of God, every time you find yourself starting to say "I AM sick," "I AM broke," "I AM not feeling well," instantly reverse this fatal condition to your progress; and declare silently with all the intensity of your being—"I AM"—which is all health, opulence, Perfection, happiness, peace, and the power to recognize Perfection in yourself and everywhere else." (9)

Emmet Fox tells us in his book, *Sermon on the Mount*, that for us to believe ourselves to be sinful is in itself to be sinful because of the consequences that will follow that thought. Jesus taught us to turn our hearts from the focus on the outer world to the focus of the inner world to connect ourselves to Creator God.

Emmet Fox talks about the story of the Rich Young Man being one of the saddest stories written because the young man missed out on the greatest opportunity in history. This story talks about the young man having great possessions, but the story goes deeper than material possessions. The story is about possessions being preconceived judgments and ideas. This story is tragic not because the young man had wealth, but because his heart was imprisoned by the love of money and his beliefs about money and material possessions.

This story is true for us today. We place importance on our appearance in the world and our knowledge about things of the world. Because we have great possessions of intellectual and spiritual pride, and great possessions of self-satisfaction, and of academic commitment, and of social prestige we are no better off than the Rich Young Man. *We are the poor in spirit.*

How can we become pure in heart so we can see God? How do we see I AM? He is not a physical, tangible being. How do we develop a spiritual perception so we can comprehend Creator God?

Heaven is within each of us. It is not some faraway place, but it is all around us and until we realize this, we will not be able to experience the love, joy, peace, and harmony of heaven.

Emmet Fox compares us with a color-blind man who lives in a world of beautiful colors in the flowers, the sky, and the colors in nature. All he sees are shades of black, gray, and white. The color-blind man does not see the clouds in the blue sky, or the life-giving green shades of the trees and he does not see the bright red of the male cardinal as it tries to attract a mate. Alas, this poor man cannot see the breathtaking colors of red, pink, yellow, and orange of a sunset or sunrise. If he were also without the sense of smell, then the garden would have no meaning for him and it is forever hidden from him.

This passage had profound new meaning for me as I recently walked through a garden nursery filled with a large variety of flowers that were red, yellow, blue, purple, just about any color you wanted to see. There was a large selection of trees and bushes all around in varying shades of green. The sweet aromas from the flowering plants were all around me lingering in the air as I was immersed in the beauty of this living creation of nature.

As I walked through the flowers and trees, I saw a blind man standing in the center of the plants. He was wearing his sunglasses to hide his eyes and he had his red-striped cane in his hands. He tapped along the pathways until he found a place to sit down as he waited for his companion to finish shopping. I wondered if he was able to smell the sweet aromas of the fragrant plants surrounding him. Or was the garden totally hidden from him?

It occurred to me that we too, are like the blind man. While we have our vision, we do not really *see* all the beauty that is around us. We can't see the "trees for the forest" so to speak. We have become blinded to our surrounding and we do not *see* God Our Father who is standing right in front of us. We have become so caught up in life, that we are not living life, we are not seeing the blessings that have been placed along our path as we walk it.

Do we feel the sensations of the textures with our fingertips of the plants encircling us? Do you feel the smoothness of the rose petals? The roughness of the peeling bark on a weeping willow? Do we feel the emotions of love, grace, peace, hope, and joy that life offers us? Or, are we blindly, emotionlessly, senselessly going through life, not experiencing life at all?

Are we like an automaton just moving through life? How sad it is for the blind man in the garden center, surrounded by all the beauty of the colors that the plants had to offer. But, it is also sadly tragic for those of us who just exist, blindly and senselessly going through life not experiencing the blessings surrounding us. We have closed ourselves off to the majesty of life itself. We have essentially become both the blind man and the rich young man at the same time. I think this story is more heartbreaking than the story of the Rich Young Man. The sad reality is we did it to ourselves. We blinded ourselves and we placed importance on the activities in life that are, in truth, nothing more than busy work. We have not only missed out on the garden, but also we have missed out on the true meaning of life. We have missed out on the Love of Our Father who created us.

The definition of "pure of heart" in this content is our subconscious mind. We accept the truth of God in the conscious mind, but it is harder to penetrate this concept into our subconscious mind. We have to take the opinion of Source, the Truth, and incorporate it into our subconscious mind for us to experience the presence of Spirit God. Until the truth is assimilated fully into the subconscious mind, it will not make any difference in our character or our life. We are literally, a "dead man walking".

Remember, "As a man thinketh in his heart, so is he." We are reminded to keep our "heart with all diligence, for out of it comes the issues of life."

As we tend to our inner thoughts, the light of these thoughts will radiate from within outward. We will become a light to the world and others will see the light coming from within us. This light illuminating from us can influence those around us. They may not know exactly what it is they are seeing, but they will sense on a higher level that your energy is of a healing source. You become the lighthouse to guide those who are trying to navigate through life's storms. Your powerful beam of light shows them where the shoreline is and keeps them from crashing into the rocks of life that can sink them and destroy them.

I once had an old man approach me while I was tending to my nursing duties in Infection Prevention at a VA Hospital tell me, "You have the 'light of God' radiating from you."

His comment both surprised and pleased me, for I had been praying for sometime that others would see the loving light of God coming from me. I had been praying that Father God's creative energy within me would be healing for the patients, staff, and others that I would come in contact with throughout the day and that they would recognize that it was God's healing light and not mine. Ask and you shall receive. This was truly a blessing for me to realize that I AM is, indeed, working within me and radiating His loving light outward. To feel the connection to the eternal stream of Love from the Universal Creator is both amazing and humbling.

As you grow in the light of God, let go of those things and people that no longer serve you. Throw out the emotions of fear, doubt, the stagnation of procrastination, and lust. Sweep out the cobwebs of attachments to the things in your life that serve no purpose in your development. Things like revenge, always wanting to be right about everything, old habits of thinking that your way is the only way to do a task, and plotting on how to make another person look foolish.

Once these things have been thrown out and swept away, fill the space within you with God's brilliant light. The warmth and love of His light will flood you and your blessings will overflow onto those around you. Feel the freedom that comes with the release of the "old" and the bringing in of the "new." As we clean out those things that no longer serve us, we begin the process of understanding that we are in control of our own soul and life. We begin to understand the laws of thought, knowing that as we learn with ever-increasing accuracy with our thought patterns, we are shaping our circumstances and our destiny.

As long as our thoughts are focused on the illusion of external circumstances, we will not be in command of the creative force that lays dormant within our mind. The soul attracts what it secretly thinks on; what it loves, and what it fears as well. It reaches to the heights of its aspirations. It plunges to the depths of its unchastened desires and these are the circumstances by which the soul receives its own.

If the focus is on the outer world of circumstances, then this is what will shape itself into our inner world of thought. It does not matter if the thoughts are of pleasurable nature or thoughts of a fearful nature, this is what we will reap. While we cannot directly choose our circumstances, we can choose and shape our thoughts, and in doing so, we indirectly shape our outward circumstances.

As you learn a new pattern of speech, speaking only in positive terms, you will see manifestations of abundance, love, joy, hope, and faith begin to appear in your life. As you give God permission to fill you with His loving light and presence you will see that you are transforming into a different being. You are becoming one with All-That-There-Is, you are created in your Father's light, you are His child created in His image.

The clue to the real purpose of life is to lose yourself to your ideas by having complete assurance in the awareness that the ideas of who or where you are, is no longer true. It is no longer the same life as it was prior to your surrender to who you now are. Your conscious speculation will determine the nature of the world in which you now live. When you ignore the current state of affairs, you then step into the desire fulfilled. Claim it and it will be realized. This is your truth in action.

There is only one truth that we have to know and that is our own truth for our life. Divine Love speaks our truth to us and all we need to know is that we are inspired by Creator to follow the path that is true to our own nature. We do not need to be concerned about another person's truth. We just need to remember that all knowledge we receive from Source leads us to our own innermost truth.

However, this door swings both ways. There are those who say that the law of attraction is Metaphysical Pseudoscience. Neil Farber MD, PhD, CLC, CPT who is a contributor to *Psychology Today* states that he disagrees with the Law of Attraction belief, "They claim material abundance and wealth are the most important manifestations to attract. The Universe sets your life purpose. You pick the specific goal based on wants; not values. This is one reason there is less passion driving goal completion because these are not deep-seated principled goals."

He goes on to say that with the law of attraction that there is no purpose, the universe determines your path to walk. There is no action that is required of one, you put the thought out there and the universe will take care of your needs. There is no plan needed because all you need to do is trust that the universe will manifest it for you. You have no date or timeline needed because it will just happen. And you have no challenges because no goals are set to achieve. We have no compassion because the negative emotions and side of life are to be avoided. Also, no support is needed since all your desires will be provided for. You can be mindless in being, in that one expects the universe to provide for you and as a result you do not need to be mindful of what is going on around you. No need to blame yourself if what you want does not materialize in your life. We blame the victim for their lot in life. We're not perfect and if you think that your life will be perfect, you are setting yourself up for disappointment. He believes that you could experience the placebo effect in your life. Last he states that, "Evidence that the LOA is an effective way of attaining goals is anecdotal, nonscientific and self-reported." In a study of about two thousand people the percentage rate of success of the law of attraction is about 0.1 percent. (18)

I am not here to dispute Dr. Farber's statements. I, in fact, encourage you to read his insightful article listed in the reference section. My intention in bringing up the topic that the law of attraction is not a legitimate resource to life is to show that there are two sides to this thought on universal supply.

Philippians 4:19: "And my God will meet all your needs according to the riches of his glory in Christ Jesus." NIV

Mt 6:8: ". . . your Father knows the things you have need of before you ask Him." NIV

Ps 34:10: ". . . those who seek the Lord shall not lack any good thing." NIV

There are numerous scriptures to support the law of attraction, but again, what happens when that is not demonstrated in one's life? Is our faith not strong enough? What is wrong with us when our needs are not met?

Let's take a look at some of the religious explanations on why prayer is not answered and why our needs are not always met.

~ Prayers are not realized when they are not according to God's will.
~ Prayers drop to the wayside when uttered in anger and seeking revenge. The prayer may be lustful and not in our best interest or in the interest of others who are involved in the situation.
~ Our prayers may not be answered when we are asking for something that we should be taking care of.
~ Prayer will go unanswered when it is a prayer uttered as a grudge.
~ Prayer is not answered when we do not expect it to be answered.

~ Prayer is not answered when we try to dictate to God on how to take care of the situation.

So, what is the right answer? All of the observations on both sides are correct to some degree. What are we supposed to think? Opinions have been stated on both sides of the doorway. Do you think that the answer could be standing somewhere in the threshold?

We are what we think. If we dwell on negative thinking such as, I feel bad, then you will feel bad. If one uses distraction therapy at times like this, they will find that by being interested in something else, such as reading a good book, it will help you feel better by taking the focus off of yourself.

Rumination (interesting word) is defined as the focused attention on the symptoms of one's distress, and on its possible causes and consequences, as opposed to its solutions. In other words, our mind gets caught in a vicious loop of constantly thinking about what is wrong with us instead of on what we can do to improve the situation.

Mainstream medicine has shown in research studies that positive thinking does have health benefits associated with it. The study of what makes life worthwhile is known as positive psychology. Is your glass half empty or half full? How well you are able to adapt to life's situations depends on your way of thinking. People who have a positive outlook on life seem to flourish and, in general, do better in life. That does not mean that they are not facing difficult situations in life or health issues at times. What it does mean is that these people are also solution-oriented to the challenges they are facing in day-to-day experiences.

According to the Mayo Clinic, positive thinking is linked to a wide range of health benefits including:

~ longer life span
~ less stress

~ lower rates of depression
~ increased resistance to the common cold
~ better stress management and coping skills
~ lower risk of cardiovascular disease-related death
~ increased physical well-being
~ better psychological health

One study of 1,558 older adults found that positive thinking could also reduce frailty during old age.

From June 7 to July 30, 1993, an experiment in meditation on the effects of the crime rate was conducted in Washington, DC. Washington was chosen because of its higher crime rate nationwide. The Transcendental Meditation (TM) technique, introduced by Maharishi Mahesh Yogi was used. It is a simple, natural, effortless procedure whereby the mind easily and naturally slips into a quieted state of thought. Once the minds of the volunteers were settled into this state of consciousness, also known as Transcendental Consciousness or pure consciousness, the experiment was begun. Volunteers came from a hundred countries to collectively meditate for long periods of time throughout the day.

The FBI had predicted in advance that with such a large-sized group there would be a certain percentage drop in violent crime. There was a twenty-seven-member independent Project Review Board consisting of sociologists and criminologists from leading universities, representatives from the police department and government that monitored its progress.

By using a time-series analysis, violent crimes were analyzed separately in terms of HRA crimes (crimes against the person) and robberies, as well as together. The maximum decrease was 23.3 percent when the size of the group of people participating was at its largest during the final week of the project.

Based on the results of the study, the steady state gain (long-term effect) associated with a permanent group of four thousand participants in the Transcendental Meditation and TM-Sidhi programs was calculated as a 48 percent reduction in HRA crimes in the District of Columbia. The results were astounding to researchers.

Nikola Tesla said it best, *"The day science begins to study non-physical phenomena, it will make more progress in one decade than in all the previous centuries of its existence. To understand the true nature of the universe, one must think in terms of energy, frequency, and vibration."*

The quantum double-slit experiment is a great example of how consciousness and our physical material world are intertwined. In this experiment, a double-slit optical system was used to test the possible role of consciousness in the collapse of the quantum wave function. This study found that factors associated with consciousness **significantly** correlated in predicted ways with perturbations in the double-slit interference pattern. (19)

Numerous experiments have been conducted over several decades by NASA, CIA, and the Defense Department on the power of the mind.

Who do you believe? The research on the Power of Positive Thinking, The Law of Attraction, or in the research that says it is all bogus? You will have to make up your own mind. For the purpose of this book, I will continue to speak from the psychological and spiritual aspect. The scientific point of view will be discussed in an upcoming book.

The point to remember is that once the conscious and subconscious minds are aligned, anything is possible.

PRAYER

I call on my Guardian Angel and the Angel of Thought. I ask that you help me align my conscious mind and subconscious mind together. Help me be like the Hind, in that, my conscious and subconscious minds are in harmony and are tracking true one to the other. Help me be aware of my thoughts at all times, to watch what I think. Help me keep my thoughts in harmony with Our Creators Loving Energy.

Amen.

13

Don't Judge Me!

We are told, "Judge not that ye be not judged. For with what judgment ye judge, ye shall be judged; and with what measure ye mete, it shall be measured to you again."

Do we truly understand these words? If we did, we would be immediately changed forever from the inside of ourselves to the outside, from top to bottom and the whole world would be changed for the better.

We judge people on how they look, how they talk, how they walk, how they interact with other people, where they live, what they do for a living; but the three top areas of judgment are on one's morality, competence, and on a person's likability.

One definition of the word judgment according to the Merriam-Webster dictionary is: 1. the process of forming an opinion or evaluation by discerning and comparing careful *judgment* of the odds 2. an opinion or estimate so formed is not worth doing in my *judgment (17)*

Another definition of judgment is a term referring to the process by which people make decisions and form conclusions based on available information and material combined with mental activity (thought) and experience.

Judgmental definition is—of, relating to, or involving judgment.

What is the difference between the two? With the word judgment you are forming an opinion on a situation or action. But, when we are being judgmental we are being critical and at times overly critical of a person.

Let's take a look at being judgmental and the damage it does to not only ourselves, but also to the people who we pass judgment on. Why is it that we invest so much time in judging others and ourselves? Do you realize that your perspective is flawed? You have only seen one side of the situation that you are passing a verdict on.

Even if the judgment is about yourself, you do not see the situation clearly. We are not honest with ourselves. We judge ourselves harshly. You do not judge yourself with compassion or love and, as a result, you are not seeing the truth in the situation.

When it comes to other people we truly don't know what they are going through. Not until we have walked in their shoes and we have seen the incident from their eyes can we understand their pain. We are wearing blinders and are being self-righteous. Your point of view is not the only valid one. When looking through a narrow viewpoint you have cut off from being objective and seeing the different possibilities of the situation. Tunnel vision is not a good thing in this instance.

What makes us so sure our point of view is right? There is our perspective, the view of the person being judged and then somewhere in the middle is the truth. Do not shove doubt aside. No one human is always right. There is no one alive who has not had to struggle in one aspect or another. Open your mind to the possibilities not seen.

Have you considered that when you are judging a person, you are most likely judging a hidden shadow side of your own personality or behavior that you do not want to admit that you have? It is painful for us to examine our shadows and more painful to admit to ourselves that we have this dark side of our psyche. Yet, to examine our weakness and inferior persona is the only way we will grow into a more complete individual.

When we judge others, we hurt them. Think about the harm that has been done to you when you have been judged by other people. It does not matter if the belief is accurate or not, the damage has been done and oftentimes cannot be repaired.

"People take different roads seeking fulfillment and happiness. Just because they're not on your road does not mean they are lost."

–Dalai Lama

How often during the course of the day do we judge? We judge the way a person chooses to dress. What color they dyed their hair. We pass judgment on how they walked into the room. We scrutinize how they talked to the waitress. We go so far as to nitpick how they go about their daily task, and on and on and on.

Our perceptions of others reveal a lot about who we are. If one is optimistic and happy, they tend to judge others as being happy and positive as well. If you are happy with your own life and are well liked by other people, you are more likely to see others as being happy with their lives and as being positive.

In contrast, if you are a negative person who is looking for fault in others, then you are more likely to see fault in others. You will only see that individual's weaknesses. You will turn a blind eye and a deaf ear to that person's assets. You will refuse to see what this person has to offer to society or what they have to offer in a personal relationship.

You will be judged in the same way you see others. Do you really understand this concept?

People tend to judge others because they fail to remember that everyone make mistakes and oftentimes we have no tolerance for mistakes. Why is it that we do not tolerate what we perceive as weakness? Individuals have differences in the ways that they seek happiness and fulfillment. This makes it hard to accept some behaviors that may seem a little out of the norm for the majority of society.

Lack of education on the disabilities that affect behavior also makes people judge others. Often when a person is struggling with mental health issues, they are judged to be dangerous or little compassion is shown to the person who is struggling with day to day challenges. They are judged to be weak both mentally and psychologically. Many times we underestimate the struggles of those individuals around us. We often underestimate the challenges of those we know well and love.

Interestingly, we tend to overestimate our struggles and challenges. We see the challenges in our lives as being more severe and more difficult to deal with than how we see the same circumstances in other people's lives. Our issues are more demanding and complicated than other people's and not easily solved. Our life is more complex and of a very sensitive nature. Other people just do not understand how difficult our life is.

Why is it that we enjoy belittling others? Our society is competitive. One wants to be on top and to be that popular person whom everyone seeks out. Everyone wants to have that charismatic personality that others are naturally drawn toward and want to follow.

We want to be this outgoing and charming person. You find that you want to be that person who everyone wants to imitate. It is interesting that people who lack confidence and a sense of who they are are often the very ones who will try to prove others wrong. Even over the smallest insignificant infraction of actions.

They are the ones who will go out of their way to point out your mistake, no matter how small it is. That individual wants to make themselves look better.

We make the assumption that everyone sees life in the same way we feel and think. This is the biggest assumption and mistake that we make. We are fearful of being ourselves around other people, because we are afraid everyone else will judge us. We fear that they will victimize us, ridicule us, and blame us, just as we have done to those around us. Guess what, that is just what they have already done. They have judged us. To protect ourselves, we reject others before they have a chance to reject us. Unfortunately that is the way of human nature.

When we are seeking change for ourselves, we sometimes feel we can be judgmental on the lives of others. We have opinions about how they should behave, about what is acceptable for them to have in their realm of existence, and how they should proceed in life. We know better what it is that they need to be doing than they do. What does that say about us? Rather judgmental, don't you think?

The fact is, how we think, speak, feel, and act toward others is how they will think, speak, feel, and act toward us. Do unto others as we would like others to do unto us. Whatever sort of behavior we direct toward others, will inevitably come back to us. Some may say, "What goes around, comes around."

The pendulum swings both ways in this mode of thinking. When we have good thoughts and act according to others, then these good thoughts and deeds will return to us in accordance. If we wish evil on others, then this too will return to us. This does not mean that the same people we have blessed or cursed will be the actual ones to return our actions. But, what it does mean is that at some point in our life, often long after we have forgotten the deed, someone else who has no knowledge of our previous actions and thoughts will repay it back to us. We will be measured by our actions point to point. (13)

A modern thought on the Golden Rule is: Think about others as you would like for them to think about you. In light of what we know to be true, the observance of this rule becomes our solemn duty to carry it out with the most earnest intent. (13)

We are gaining a new understanding, a new concept of the great law of the Golden Rule and how it works. In this understanding is it possible to rise above this Great Law in the name of THE CHRIST?

We seem to think that the term "Christ" is identical with Jesus, the individual, but is it? It is not. Christ is a technical term that can be defined as the Absolute Spiritual Truth about anything. To know the Truth about a person, or condition, or circumstance, will immediately heal that person, or condition, or circumstance to the degree that this Truth is understood by the thinker. This is the center of spiritual healing. Whenever the Christ, the True Idea, is lifted up in thought, healing begins whether it be physical, emotional, mental, or spiritual.(13)

We should claim this Divine Intelligence for any person or situation and realize that God is the soul of mankind. Because the Christ is nothing less than the direct action of Father God Himself, the Self-knowing of Spirit, overrides everything else.(13)

This higher law of Spirit overshadows everything. It overshadows all of the lower laws of the physical and mental dimensions. We know the Law of Karma forgets nothing and is actually a law for matter and mind only. It is not a law for Spirit. God is perfect and eternal, is unchangingly good. In our Father the Judge, there is no bad Karma to be reaped. Bad karma cannot be sown. When we pray or meditate and transfer our attention to Him, we come under the law of perfect Good, and Karma is destroyed. (13)

We have the choice of Karma or Christ. This is the greatest news for us. We *have* the choice. We have *free will*. We can remain in the realm of mind and matter bound by Karma, or we can pray in the Realm of Spirit; the Christ and be free. We have the choice, Christ or Karma. CHRIST IS LORD OF KARMA. (13)

Will any mistake, any horrendous sin, be erased from the Book of Life? Will all of its punishment and suffering naturally accruing to it, be wiped clean? Yes, of course it is erased. There is no evil that the Healing Christ will not destroy. There is no evil that can't be healed.(13)

We must not think that the consequences of our actions are to be evaded by prayer. We must not think that a prayer with little thought given behind the action of our deeds will wipe out the natural consequences. No superficial prayer will rectify the sin or punishment that will follow. But, with sufficient realization of God's character, we know that He can fundamentally alter the character of the sinner. His character is needed in order to wipe clean the punishment that otherwise will follow the sin. When sufficient prayer and repentance have been made, we become a changed person. One will have no desire to repeat their misdeed. We are then saved and our transactions are remitted, for Christ is Lord of Karma.

Another misconception is the false belief that we have to do something to meet the requirements to enter into the Love of God. We are told that we are born into sin and that we are sinful. Many religions teach that it doesn't matter how good we are or not, we still will not measure up.

But, how is it determined if a person can measure up or not? We are taught that we can enter into the Kingdom of God by His grace alone. If this is true, then Creator is the only one who says if we meet the requirements of salvation or not.

In our erroneous way of thinking, we think if God judges then we too can judge others as well. We rush to view others who are supposed to be righteous as being perfect in the sight of God. Anyone with even the slightest imperfection has been condemned to hell.

When we deem others as righteous or imperfect, we have placed ourselves in a deadly trap of our own doing. In doing so, we are unable to be released from the condemnation we have placed on others and ourselves.

Through the years, the Lord's Prayer has been rewritten in a style that is more in keeping with modern culture. In doing so, they have diluted the true meaning of the words in the Lord's Prayer. We tend to recite the Lord's Prayer without thinking about the true meaning of the words. It becomes repetition and Jesus teaches us to pray with meaning and understanding. There are many books written on the Lord's Prayer, so I will not go into a discussion on the meaning of the Lord's Prayer at this time.

Jesus taught us to pray in the affirmative form of prayer to be used for all healing work. We have been taught that the supplicatory prayer in which we beg and whine and plead to God as if we were children is always wrong. So, how should we pray?

The highest form of prayer is one of true contemplation, in which the thought of the Eternal and our thought become one. This is the unity that is rarely experienced. Pray in whatever way you find the easiest. For the easiest way is the best. Talk *with* God, not *at* Him. Whisper the words that are in your heart, using your own sincere words in communing with Creator God. Remember, that our brain does not do the thinking, but our heart is where our true thoughts come from. The brain knows nothing, but the heart knows everything.

In prayer, we have to track our conscious mind true with our subconscious mind. Prayer is the art of believing what is defined by the senses, and is dealt almost entirely with the subconscious. The subconscious mind will fully accept what the conscious mind places into it. The thoughts and feeling locked into the beliefs that are imprinted within the mind will charge it with a mission that will be fully executed.

There can be no conflict in your mind when you pray. Know that the desire of the heart will be completed by the law of universal attraction and God's love for us.

Let's take a look at the conscious mind, the subconscious mind, and the superconsciousness of our higher self.

In defining consciousness, we learn it means: 1. the state of being conscious; awareness. 2. the thoughts and feelings, collectively, of an individual or of an aggregate of people. 3. full activity of the mind and senses, as in waking life: to regain consciousness.

Your subconscious is the part of your mind that can influence you or affect your behavior even though you are not aware of it.

The superconscious mind is that which is beyond both the conscious and subconscious minds, reaching into the highest level of awareness. It is the universal mind that is at one with Brahman, which is also the source of intuition. The physical center of the superconscious mind is the brain's frontal lobe between the eyebrows. Some call it the third eye.

As we have discussed, it is imperative that the conscious and subconscious minds are aligned. How do we align our conscious and subconscious minds? What steps do we need to take to stay positive in our outlook on life?

The function of your subconscious mind is to store and retrieve information. Your subconscious mind is subjective. It does not think or reason independently; it merely obeys the commands it receives. The subconscious mind causes you to feel emotionally and physically uncomfortable whenever you attempt to do anything new or different. It will try to prevent you from changing any of your established patterns of behavior. It does not like the unknown and will strive to keep your behavior patterns the same. Like a child, it will try to manipulate you.

The subconscious mind is the guardian or the gatekeeper, using the information stored from these events to deduct likely probabilities and prompt us into action accordingly. It is the gateway to access our Higher Conscious. Most of us believe that we make decisions based on our conscious mind. However, the truth is, your subconscious mind is the primary motivator behind every decision you make. It really is the boss. The subconscious is where everything that has consciously or unconsciously happened to you has been stored. It holds all your experiences that you have had throughout your life; good and bad. This is how you are influenced, how you go through life, what motivates you to do what you do. It holds the rules and regulations that you have imposed on yourself and directs you on how you will automatically get through your day.

Your subconscious mind can pick up messages much quicker than your conscious mind. It can process information five hundred thousand times faster than what the conscious mind can. Impressive, isn't it? So, even a quick glance at the store's display window you just passed could have resulted in the display being stored in your subconscious. And that message can influence later decisions that impact your life. You can be drawn to go back to that store when you are ready to make a purchase.

When you become aware of a habit or belief that is affecting your life negatively, you can consciously make a choice to change this pattern of thinking. To do this, you need to start adding positive messages to your subconscious mind that will help you achieve the desired results. To change your habits, you consciously decide to take in new ideas and thoughts and let them sink into your subconscious mind until they become beliefs. Remember, we are what we continue to think about. The more we think about an idea, the faster it will integrate into our subconscious mind and become a reality.

What are some of the tools we need to accomplish our desires? How do we go about reaching this desired goal? Can we reach our goals?

1. Close your eyes and take a few deep breaths from the diaphragm. Then focus your attention behind your eyelids. When you find yourself trapped in that compulsive loop of negative thinking, breath into it. Bring your focus back to the moment. Acknowledge the compulsive thoughts

and focus on your desired thoughts. Shift your thought process to the desired outcomes.

2. Bring your focus into balance by connecting to the energy of the earth. Our bodies are designed to be in synchronization with the rhythm of the earth to maintain health. This activity helps you to center your thought process and ground you to the earth. Imagine that you feel the energy of the earth coming up through your feet. Feel your energy extending into the earth, growing deeper into the earth like roots from a tree. Feel the divine energy coming into the crown of your head gently spiraling down to meet the energy of the earth as it slowly begins to rise up through your feet into your solar plexus and then into your heart. Both of these energies will intermingle at the heart. You will notice a difference in awareness right away with this exercise. You feel more powerful than you do when you are lost in your compulsive thought process. You feel more present and aware of what is really happening around you. You are more in control of what you are focused on and thinking about.

3. Imagine the positive outcome of your heart's desires. Visualize the desired outcome as already happened. Bring it into the present time.

4. Turn off the negative Monkey Chatter. Eliminate the negative influences in your life. They serve no purpose in you reaching your goals. It is important to avoid the people around you who are making you think negative thoughts. As long as you are around them, your thoughts are going to stay focused on their negative energy. The negative people who are in your life will influence you to have negative thoughts and it will be harder to change your thoughts into positive thought waves.

5. Focus on what is and not what if. Stay in the present moment. Do not allow your mind to wander into the imaginary world of "what if".

6. Remember, "This too shall pass." Nothing stays the same. Understanding that nothing is permanent will help you change your perspective from negative thoughts to positive thoughts instantly. Realizing that good things do happen will help you manifest positive outcomes and feel more grounded and positive in the present moment.

7. Silence the negative internal chatter. Become aware that you are experiencing negative feedback. Then bring yourself back to the present moment. Develop staying in the moment and not letting your mind wander into the realm of negative thoughts.

8. Stay in the present moment. Stay in reality. Do a reality check when you notice that your mind has wandered off track. Practice mindfulness by paying attention to what it is that you are actually doing.

9. Write down positive affirmations. Tell yourself positive aspects about who you are. Write down what you have accomplished during the day. It does not matter how small the achievement was. Making the bed in the morning is an accomplishment.

10. You are your own best friend. Remember that! Learn to think only positive thoughts about yourself. Be your own cheerleader! This is not self-centeredness, it is a healthy respect of who you are.

We think that our conscious mind is in control, it is not. The subconscious mind is in charge. It is the gatekeeper and sometimes things can slip by when the gatekeeper is distracted. It takes in all the information that we receive throughout the day. We do not have to become helpless victims of our thoughts. We have the power to control our thoughts and be the masters of our lives.

The reason most people fail to become the masters of their own mind is because they do not know how the Subconscious Mind works. Since our desires come from our Subconscious mind, it is essential to know the differences between the subconscious and the conscious minds.

The subconscious mind thinks in the present only. It does not distinguish between good or bad, positive or negative. It takes in information at face value. It does not filter out what is imagined and what is real. We are what we think. You will see this statement many times. I am trying to impress upon you the importance in paying attention to your thoughts. From the moment an action becomes a habit, the subconscious executes it automatically.

While your Conscious mind is your logical, rational, analytical mind, your Subconscious mind is your illogical, irrational, and nonanalytical mind. It believes ANYTHING and EVERYTHING whether it makes logical sense or not. It believes what you tell it, no questions asked. When you try to accomplish goals through your conscious mind it takes time to integrate them into your life. But, working through your Subconscious mind and making it believe you have already attained your goals, you have hastened the process of seeing your heart's desires coming into fruition. Seldom do we use conscious thinking in making our decisions. Most decisions are based on our approach or avoidance reactions that occur before conscious awareness is set into action. Once activated, the subconscious mind targets the goals it perceives that are to be fulfilled.

Your subconscious mind is connected with Divine Knowledge. Christians may refer to this energy as the Holy Spirit, or the creative energy known as God, the Beginning and the End. In Vedic teachings, this energy is Known as the Supreme Being. This energy uses karma as connection from one lifetime to the next, and one soul to another. Today, many refer to this energy as "The Universe." The subconscious mind is always connected with this energy source known as Divine Creation.

The subconscious is in constant communication to our Higher Consciousness. It is this connection of the subconscious to the Creator Source, which is programmed to reward us with the very things we dwell on in our thoughts. The subconscious mind always gravitates to what is familiar, not what is best for you. The unknown is resisted by the subconscious because it cannot see all the variables to predict an outcome. The subconscious mind is not able to see the possibilities, so it is necessary to use the conscious mind to inject new ideas by asking questions and examining the possibilities along with the outcomes of these new ideas.

The more we work with our subconscious mind and stay connected to our higher conscious mind, the easier it is to balance our health mentally, physically, emotionally, and spiritually.

It is important to align our subconscious beliefs with our conscious ones if we wish to achieve fulfillment in all areas of our life. By using techniques like hypnosis and guided meditation, we can tame, empower, and program the subconscious mind to be our protector by guiding and directing our life to obtain our unlimited potential and to realize our heart's true desires and dreams.

One interesting aspect about the subconscious is that, when you sleep, it builds a powerful creative bridge connecting thoughts that you had in a conscious state to the thoughts you have during sleep so when you wake it will make that reconnection between the two.

The subconscious mind is essential for us to function. Our conscious mind is not able to comprehend many different thoughts at the same time, usually only one thought at a time. Most of our thinking activities take place in the subconscious mind. This is where we connect with our intuition and inner knowing that connects us with Spirit Most High.

Intuition works behind the scenes collecting our past experiences and learning. It gives us the ability to understand something immediately without the need for conscious reasoning. Our insights, our intuitions reflect those things which we know or consider likely from instinctive feeling rather than conscious reasoning. Inner knowing is the mind's connection with our spiritual energy. It has access to universal knowledge and reflects our true nature to Creator who shows unconditional love. From our inner knowing, we see things from a viewpoint of empathy, compassion, understanding, and love. Intuition does not make logical arguments, it just accepts what we believe to be the truth; whether it is a truth or a lie. The more in tune you are with your subconscious, the closer you will be to breaking through to understanding how the conscious and subconscious minds work together. The intelligence of your subconscious mind is infinitely far more than all the intelligence of your conscious mind.

"Remember that your dominating thoughts attract, through a definite law of nature, by the shortest and most convenient route, their physical counterpart. Be careful what your thoughts dwell upon."

—Napolean Hill

Guilty Prayers, we do not have to pray them once we realize that we have a choice to pray in a higher dimension, in the realm of our Lord God, our Creator and Father. Once our prayers become like the feet of the hind, our conscious and subconscious minds tracking true one to the other, then we have reached the top of the mountain and nothing can prevent us from knowing God and being known by Him.

Now we have experienced "The Shift."

PRAYER

I pray that this book has been an inspiration for you. I pray that within this book you have found some tools to help you along your journey in life. Blessings and peace to you as you travel through this lifetime of experiences and through this school of life.

So it is said, so it is done.

References

1. http://www.gateways-to-inner-peace.com/dealing-with-guilt.html
2. Understanding the Male Temperament: Tim LaHaye . . . https://www.amazon.com/Understanding-Male-Temperament-Tim-LaHaye/
3. Learning to Forgive: The 5-Steps of Forgiveness July 27, 2008 by Anthony Centore
4. http://gailbrenner.com/2012/01/10-life-changing-facts-about-anger/. 10 Life-Changing Facts About Anger Posted By: Gail Brenner
5. https://www.mayoclinic.org/diseases-conditions/post-traumatic-stress-disorder/symptoms-causes/syc-20355967
6. Home/Relationships/How to Deal With Rejection in Love—When He Doesn't Love You Back http://psychologia.co/how-to-deal-with-rejection/
7. Self-blame: The Ultimate Emotional Abuse. Michael J. Formica, MS, MA, EdM
8. The Self-Blame Game: An Obstacle to Change By Jonice Webb, PhD
9. The "I AM" Discourses (St. Germain Series) volume 3, "I AM" ACTIVITY of St. Germain Foundation; www

.SAINTGERMAINFOUNDATION.org; www
.SAINTGERMAINpress.com

10. Parenting Truth: You Are Not to Blame for Your Child's
Behavior By Kim Abraham, LMSW & Marney Studaker-
Cordner, LMSWhttps://www.empoweringparents.com/
article/parenting-truth-you-are-not-to-blame-for-your-
childs-behavior/

11. The Secrets of Successful Prayer. Selections from Sefer
Ba'al Shem Tov Parashat Noah—Amud HaTefilah

12. I Will Lift Up Mine Eyes by Glenn Clark. Published by
Harper & Row 1937

13. The Sermon On The Mount: The Key to Success in Life
by Emmet Fox. Published by Harper Collins e-books,
Copyright 1934 by Emmet Fox.

14. https://www.nami.org/Learn-More/Mental-Health-
Conditions/Depression

15. https://en.wikipedia.org/wiki/Regret

16. https://www.healthtopia.net/disease/mental-health/phobia/
philophobia-fear-of-love

17. https://www.merriam-webster.com/dictionary/judgment

18. Neil Farber MD, PhD., CLC, CPT, The Blame Game,
The Truth About the Law of Attraction It doesn't exist!,
Posted Sep 18, 2016

19. Science Proves That Human Consciousness and Our
Material World Are Intertwined: See For Yourself,
Published March 8, 2014 By Arjun Walia

20. Source: http://spdrdng.com/posts/conscious-vs-
subconscious-processing

21. THE DIVINE THE SCIENTIFIC CURE FOR DEPRES-
SION: PRAYER. Exclusive: Hanne Nabintu Herland shares
studies proving mental, physical benefits

22. Dr. Lisa Miller—Clinical Psychologist and Spirituality.
https://www.macmillanspeakers.com/lisamiller

About the Author

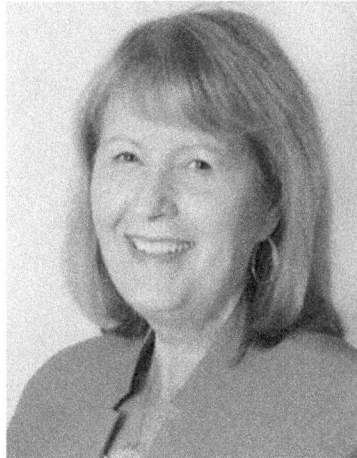

My career started as a LPN. I then received an Associate in Science in Nursing or RN. The RN evolved into a B.S.N. and before I knew it I was earning a Master's in Health Care Administration while simultaneously earning a Ph.D. in Natural Health. Along the way I received certification in Therapeutic Hypnosis and advanced certification in Regression Hypnosis.

In 2017, I was hit by a semi-truck ending my nursing career. Nursing is not my only passion. My passion is giving people the tools they need for better health.

I've taken the knowledge I've gained through the years to help individuals, just like yourself, by putting this information into books. My years as a VA nurse, working in the mental health clinic, gave me an insight into the struggles people have on a daily basis with emotional issues.

It's my sincerest desire for *Guilty Prayers* to be the tool you use for better mental health!

Life is not measured by the number of breaths we take, but by the moments that take our breath away.
—AUTHOR UNKNOWN

Visit Janet's blog: *mindbodyconnectionhypnosis.com*